Testosterone - Functions, Uses, Deficiencies, and Substitution

Edited by Hirokazu Doi

Published in London, United Kingdom

Testosterone - Functions, Uses, Deficiencies, and Substitution
http://dx.doi.org/10.5772/intechopen.102212
Edited by Hirokazu Doi

Contributors
Hirokazu Doi, Zied Kaabia, Oyovwi Mega Obukohwo, Nwangwa Eze Kingsley, Ovuakporaye Irikefe Simon, Emojevwe Victor, Okoro Ogheneyebrorue Godswill, Rotu Arientare Rume, Ben-Azu Benneth, Onome Bright Oghenetega, Patrick Godwin Okwute, Falajiki Y. Faith, Kenneth W.K. Ho, Nidia N. Gomez, Verónica S. Biaggio, Eloy Salinas, María Verónica Pérez Chaca, María Eugenia Ciminari, Silvina Mónica Alvarez, Silvana N. Piquillem

First published in London, United Kingdom, 2023 by IntechOpen
IntechOpen is the global imprint of INTECHOPEN LIMITED, registered in England and Wales, registration number: 11086078, 5 Princes Gate Court, London, SW7 2QJ, United Kingdom

British Library Cataloguing-in-Publication Data
A catalogue record for this book is available from the British Library

Additional hard and PDF copies can be obtained from orders@intechopen.com

Testosterone - Functions, Uses, Deficiencies, and Substitution
Edited by Hirokazu Doi
p. cm.
Print ISBN 978-1-83969-975-7
Online ISBN 978-1-83969-976-4
eBook (PDF) ISBN 978-1-83969-977-1

Meet the editor

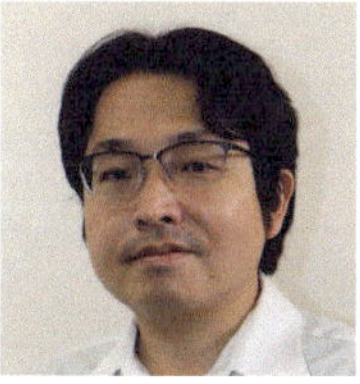

Hirokazu Doi is an Associate Professor of Information and Management Systems Engineering at Nagaoka University of Technology, Japan, and a specially appointed associate professor in the Data Science and AI Innovation Research Promotion Center, Shiga University, Japan. His main research topics include cognitive and neural mechanisms of human social perception and decision-making. He is also engaged in the development of supplementary diagnostics systems for psychiatric conditions and data-driven analysis of neural activation patterns.

Contents

Preface

Testosterone exerts varying effects on the physiological function and morphology of biological organisms at multiple stages of life. Thus, elucidation of mechanisms underlying development and sexual differentiation in many species, including humans, requires in-depth knowledge about the functions of testosterone. Research into testosterone leads to novel insights in medical and natural sciences as well as social sciences. By utilizing the knowledge from basic research on testosterone function, researchers can also develop novel ways to exploit its potential for therapeutic purposes. This book includes contributions from interdisciplinary fields, including internal medicine, molecular biology, veterinary medicine, and evolutionary psychology. It describes what is currently known about the androgenic function and its underlying mechanisms using state-of-the-art analytical techniques. Some chapters deal with the ethical and safety issues surrounding the clinical and practical application of achievements in testosterone research. I hope that readers will gain broad perspectives on the biology and function of testosterone and understand the diversity of academic fields impacted by incorporating insights from testosterone research.

Hirokazu Doi
Department of Information and Management Systems Engineering,
Nagaoka University of Technology,
Nagaoka City, Niigata Prefecture, Japan

Section 1

Basics of Testosterone

Chapter 1

Introductory Chapter: Broad Impact of Testosterone Research

Hirokazu Doi

1. Introduction

Physiological functions in animals and humans undergo many developmental changes throughout their lifespans. During the fetal period, functional structures of organs are formed, and they undergo maturational changes at multiple developmental stages after birth.

The effects of androgens are broadly classified as organizational and activational affects [1, 2]. Organizational effects refer to the function of androgens in the formation and sexual differentiation of organs, mainly during the prenatal period and puberty. Biologically available androgens exert phasic effects on physiological functions through their activational effect. Organizational effects partly determine the sensitivity of tissues to androgens. Thus, the organizational and activational effects of androgens interact to influence an organism's bodily functions and behavioral patterns.

Testosterone significantly contributes to maturational changes in physiological functions and is the primary determinant of sexually dimorphic traits. Thus, it is crucial in describing the functions and behaviors of organisms to understand how testosterone functions at each stage of development. Considering this, it is natural that testosterone has been and will continue to be the focus of interest for scholars in many academic fields. Here are some examples of disciplines that benefit from the knowledge of testosterone functionality.

1. Owing to the diversity of androgenic functions, deficiency or excess testosterone leads to various malfunctions. The highly prevalent conditions of osteoporosis [3], reduced libido, erectile dysfunction [4], and depression [5] have been linked to testosterone deficiency. Therefore, ameliorating the symptoms derived from hypergonadism or hypogonadism is an important theme in many branches of medical research.

2. Androgens facilitate sexual differentiation and modulate the central nervous system functions. Behavioral endocrinology studies have consistently revealed the role of testosterone in controlling mating and parenting behaviors in wide range of species, including rodents, avians, and humans [6]. In addition, psychologists have revealed an association between peripheral testosterone levels and individual differences in personality and psychological traits such as aggression and impulsivity [7]. Several researchers have argued that the degree of masculinization induced by prenatal exposure to androgens partly determines the cognitive

style and can cause autism spectrum disorders [8]. Thus, in addition to medical and natural sciences, studies on androgenic functions have implications for humanity and the social sciences as well.

2. Relevance of investigation into androgenic function to many research fields

It is difficult to elucidate the functionality of testosterone and the precise mechanism by which it exerts its effects on testosterone. There are several reasons for the difficulties in studying androgen function and its underlying mechanisms. Testosterone modulates and controls physiological functions in combination with other hormones. Therefore, researchers must carefully exclude confounding variables to avoid spurious associations between the phenotype of interest and androgens. Second, there are multiple pathways through which androgens influence target tissues. For example, testosterone and its metabolite, dihydrotestosterone, bind to the androgen receptor, thereby inducing genomic effect on target cell function [9]. Alternatively, testosterone influences cell function indirectly through aromatization to estradiol [10]. Such complexity in an androgenic pathway makes it even more difficult for researchers to narrow down the critical steps to implement effective clinical and practical interventions targeting androgenic functions.

A large amount of knowledge has accumulated about androgenic function, and its underlying mechanisms, and analytical techniques. It should not be overlooked either to consider how to implement regulatory systems that oversee the ethical and safety issues surrounding the practical application of the findings from basic research.

It is beneficial for researchers and practitioners alike in various fields such as internal medicine, molecular biology, veterinary medicine, and evolutionary psychology to gain broad perspectives on the biology and function of testosterone and understand the diversity of academic fields impacted by incorporating insights from testosterone research.

Author details

Hirokazu Doi
Department of Information and Management Systems Engineering, Nagaoka University of Technology, Nagaoka City, Niigata Prefecture, Japan

*Address all correspondence to: hdoi_0407@yahoo.co.jp

References

[1] Arnold AP, Breedlove SM. Organizational and activational effects of sex steroids on brain and behavior: A reanalysis. Hormones and Behavior. 1985;**19**(4):469-498

[2] Schulz KM, Sisk CL. The organizing actions of adolescent gonadal steroid hormones on brain and behavioral development. Neuroscience & Biobehavioral Reviews. 2016;**70**:148-158

[3] Golds G, Houdek D, Arnason T. Male hypogonadism and osteoporosis: The effects, clinical consequences, and treatment of testosterone deficiency in bone health. International Journal of Endocrinology. 2017;**2017**:4602129

[4] Tsujimura A. The relationship between testosterone deficiency and men's health. The World Journal of Men's Health. 2013;**31**(2):126-135

[5] Almeida OP, Yeap BB, Hankey GJ, Jamrozik K, Flicker L. Low free testosterone concentration as a potentially treatable cause of depressive symptoms in older men. Archives of General Psychiatry. 2008;**65**(3):283-289

[6] Zilioli S, Bird BM. Functional significance of men's testosterone reactivity to social stimuli. Frontiers in Neuroendocrinology. 2017;**47**:1-18

[7] Batrinos ML. Testosterone and aggressive behavior in man. International Journal of Endocrinology and Metabolism. 2012;**10**(3):563-568

[8] Baron-Cohen S. The extreme male brain theory of autism. Trends in Cognitive Sciences. 2002;**6**(6):248-254

[9] Davey RA, Grossmann M. Androgen receptor structure, function and biology: From bench to bedside. The Clinical Biochemist. Reviews. 2016;**37**(1):3-15

[10] Purves-Tyson TD, Arshi MS, Handelsman DJ, Cheng Y, Keast JR. Androgen and estrogen receptor-mediated mechanisms of testosterone action in male rat pelvic autonomic ganglia. Neuroscience. 2007;**148**(1):92-104

Chapter 2

Testosterone: The Male Sex Hormone

Oyovwi Mega Obukohwo, Ben-Azu Benneth, Ovuakporaye Irikefe Simon, Onome Bright Oghenetega, Emojevwe Victor, Falajiki Y. Faith, Patrick Godwin Okwute, Rotu Arientare Rume, Okoro Ogheneyebrorue Godswill and Nwangwa Eze Kingsley

Abstract

Males primarily use testosterone as a sex hormone. Through its effects on the androgen receptor, it is released by the interstitial cells of the testes and is in charge of the male external genitalia development as well as the internal reproductive glands and ducts during adolescence and maturity. Additionally, testosterone is required for the descent of testes via the inguinal canal in the last 2 months of fetal development. When a Y chromosome and consequently the SRY gene are missing from an embryo, ovaries form. The Wolffian ducts do not mature because the fetal ovaries do not release enough testosterone. It is mostly used to treat male hypogonadism. Notably, this chapter addresses the following context: historical view of testosterone research, biosynthesis, secretion, metabolism, transport mechanism, biological actions, health benefit of testosterone, factors that promote and inhibit testosterone secretion, therapeutic implication as well as pathophysiology of testosterone secretion.

Keywords: testosterone, Leydig cell, sex hormone-binding globulin, GnRH, aromatase, cytochrome P450, 5-alpha reductase

1. Introduction

Testosterone as one of the major male hormone, is in charge of governing the development of male sex traits, spermatogenesis, and fertility [1]. The fetus first experiences the effects of testosterone. The initial 6 weeks of development result in identical male and female reproductive tissues. The Y chromosomes SRY (sex-related gene) drives the development of the testicles during week 7 of pregnancy. From sertoli cells in the testis cords, seminiferous tubules are produced (fetal testicles). The upper part of the vaginal canal, uterus, and fallopian tubes all regress as a result of a Müllerain inhibitory substance (MIS) secreted by the Sertoli cells (Müllerian structures normally present in women).

2. Historical view of testosterone research

Scientists of Ancient days knew that removal of the testicle would take away the vitality and aggression of men and beast. Historically, castration (removal of testes) was performed on male slaves who guarded Muslim harems. It was also used on some male singers during boyhood to preserve a high pitched voice. The testicles are male gonads, or sex gland, that produces sperm and secret androgens. The production of androgens by the testes is controlled by certain pituitary hormones called gonadotropins. Testosterone, or the male sex hormone, is the most significant and active hormone. Testosterone is mostly produced in the testes, although it is also produced in minor amounts in the adrenal glands and the female ovaries.

According to Freeman et al. [2], testosterone's origins and effects have been understood throughout human history.

In 1934, David et al. [3] was the first to isolate testosterone molecule and its structure and this won him a Noble Prize in 1935.

In 1938, the beneficial effect of testosterone on impaired glucose tolerance was discovered by Kenyon [4].

In 1939, a famous Scientist called Heinrich Schumann found it to improve intermittent claudication and reduce angina pectoris, as well as confirming it to cure gangrene [5].

In 1945, another scientist called Waldman [6] showed its function to stop angina pectoris.

Hamwi [7] demonstrated in 1951 that testosterone can enhance nitrogen balance and boost lean muscle hypertrophy.

In 1960s, another scientist discovered it can lower cholesterol as confirmed by Hartgens and Kuipers [8].

In 1962, scientists called Katz and Katz [9] normalized the abnormal electrocardiograms of 2000 cardiac patients with synthetic testosterone.

It can help with diabetic retinopathy, according to a 1963 research by Lawrence et al. [10].

According to Kim et al. [11], scientists first discovered that testosterone can reduce diabetic patients' need for insulin and their body fat percentage in 1964.

The Columbia University Department of Medicine stated in May 1994 that low levels of free testosterone are a risk factor and directly correspond with the severity of coronary artery disease in men [12].

2.1 Biosynthesis of testosterone

The 500 million Leydig cells, which account for about 5% of the mature testis' volume and are situated in the interstitial region of the testis between the seminiferous tubules, use an enzymatic process to convert cholesterol into testosterone. The most common method is the de novo synthesis of cholesterol from acetate, but preformed cholesterol can also be received from an external source, including circulating low-density lipoproteins, or intracellular cholesterol ester storage [13].

Two multifunctional cytochrome P450 complexes are required for the production of 17-hydroxylase/17,20 lyase (CYP17A1 or P450c17, which hydroxylates the C17 and C18 side chains) and cholesterol side-chain cleavage (CYP11A1 or P450scc, which produces C20 and C22 hydroxylation and C20,22 lyase activity) [13]. The regulation of 17,20 lyase activity, which is active in the gonads but inactive in the adrenals and is independent of 17-hydroxylase activity, is tissue-specific and a critical fork in the steroidogenic pathways. The enzyme cofactors that have the greatest impact on the directionality of the route flux are cytochrome b5 and the membrane-bound flavoprotein P450 oxidoreductase (POR), which serves a variety of functions as a reductase. One protein with several functions houses both functions [14]. Adrenal androgens do, however, make a far bigger proportionate contribution to the circulating testosterone in women than it does to the testosterone circulating in men [15]. Additionally, it has been reported that the weak adrenal androgen precursor DHEA can be used to produce some extragonadal testosterone and dihydrotestosterone [16]. In the mitochondria of Leydig cells, LH regulates the rate-limiting conversion of cholesterol to pregnenolone, which in turn regulates the release of testicular testosterone. The inner mitochondrial membrane is home to the cytochrome P450 cholesterol side-chain cleavage enzyme complex, which mediates this process. Proteins like sterol carrier protein 2 [17] control the transfer of cholesterol to mitochondrial steroidogenic enzymes. This facilitates the transfer of cholesterol from the cytoplasm to the mitochondria along with steroidogenic acute regulatory protein [18] and translocator protein [19], which control cholesterol transport across the mitochondrial membrane. The following enzyme activity is present in the endoplasmic reticulum of the Leydig cell. Despite the fact that the precise physical process that leads to such high intratesticular testosterone and related steroid concentrations in the testis is still unknown, the high testicular testosterone production rate produces both high local concentrations of testosterone (up to 1 g/g tissue, which is roughly 100 times higher than blood concentrations) and rapid turnover of testosterone (200 times per day) [20].

2.2 Secretion of testosterone

In order to maintain male virilization, testosterone is secreted intermittently during the first trimester of intrauterine life (coinciding with the differentiation of the masculine genital tract), as the perinatal androgen surge (with as-yet-undetermined physiologic significance), and continuously after puberty. The sudden increases in testosterone output from the testicles, which rise roughly 30-fold over levels found in prepubertal toddlers, women, or castrate men, are what caused the dramatic physical changes associated with male puberty. After middle age, circulating testosterone levels gradually decline and gonadotrophin and sex hormone-binding globulin (SHBG) levels rise [21], with these tendencies being missing until late old age in men who remain in great health [22], but exaggerated by the presence of chronic illness [23]. Additionally, there are temporal trends, such as an increase in obesity prevalence [24] and variations in testosterone immunoassays due to artifactual methods that differ from standard mass spectrometry-based assessments [25].

Leydig cell attrition and malfunction, as well as atherosclerosis of testicular arteries, are all functionally responsible for these age-related alterations brought on by the chronic disease accumulation [26]. Meanwhile, the ageing of the hypothalamic-pituitary-testicular complex gradually functions abnormally on several levels, which together cause men to age with reduced levels of circulating testosterone [26]. Testosterone leaves the testis by diffusing into the bloodstream across cell membranes, similar to other lipophilic steroids synthesized by steroidogenic tissues. Smaller amounts also get to the fluid in the tubules and lymphatics. After puberty, males synthesize over 95% of the testosterone found in their blood by testicular secretion; the remaining 5% is created through extragonadal conversion of precursors such dehydroepiandrosterone and androstenedione, which have relatively low intrinsic androgenic potencies. The liver, kidney, muscle, and adipose tissue are only a few extragonadal tissues that can convert these weak androgens, which are primarily produced by the adrenal cortex, into bioactive sex steroids.

Endogenous adrenal androgens play a much smaller role in men's direct virilization than they do in women. Moreover, androgen-sensitive prostate cancer is not significantly affected biologically by remaining androgens in the blood and tissues following pharmacological or surgical castration. Although peripheral interconversion of adrenal androgen precursors and direct gonadal secretion account for roughly equal amounts of blood testosterone, adrenal androgens are proportionally more responsible for the significantly lower levels of circulating testosterone (5% of men) in children and women [15]. Exogenous dehydroepiandrosterone cannot produce enough blood testosterone to replace male androgens at physiologic replacement dosages of 50 mg/day when supplied orally to humans [27]. It also does not elicit dose-dependent increases in circulating estradiol in males.

Calculating the pace at which hormones are produced can be done using the metabolic clearance rate, mean blood levels of testosterone, testicular arteriovenous differences, and testicular blood flow rate (from bolus injection or steady-state isotope infusion utilizing high-specific-activity tracers). These methods accurately estimate a testosterone production rate of 3–10 mg/day under steady-state settings using tritiated [28] or non-radioactive deuterated [29] tracers with interconversion rates of around 4% to dihydrotestosterone (DHT) [28] and 0.2% to estradiol (hours to days). The factors that these methods, which are oversimplified and focus on steady-state conditions, ignore include postural influences on hepatic blood flow, episodic variability in circulating testosterone levels over shorter time periods (minutes to hours), pulsatile LH secretion, and diurnal periodicity [30]. The primary elements that are known to affect the metabolic clearance rate of testosterone are circulating SHBG concentration, diurnal rhythm, and postural effects on hepatic blood flow [29]. Significant genetic [31] and environmental [29] factors have been proven to have an impact on testosterone levels. Variations in SHBG reduce the severity of these effects.

3. Mechanism of testosterone secretion

During puberty, the hypothalamic-pituitary-gonadal axis controls gonadotropin levels and gonad function. LH and follicle-stimulating hormone are also secreted by the anterior pituitary, which receives GnRH from the brain via the hypothalamohypophyseal portal system (FSH). Two gonadotropic hormones called LH and FSH act on gonad receptors while moving through the bloodstream. Through its effects on the Leydig cells, LH in particular promotes the generation of testosterone. By using negative feedback, testosterone controls its own secretion. High blood testosterone concentrations impair the anterior pituitary's ability to respond to GnRH stimuli and reduce hypothalamic GnRH release [1]. Throughout the reproductive lifetimes of males, the hypothalamus pulses GnRH every 1–3 h. From the onset of puberty, when levels start to rise, until the third decade of life, when levels peak and gradually start to fall, average plasma levels of FSH and LH stay largely constant in spite of this pulsatile release. Poor testosterone levels prior to puberty are an indication of low gonadotropin and GnRH production. The production of GnRH increases noticeably throughout puberty as a result of changes in the neuronal input to the hypothalamus and changes in brain activity.

Cholesterol is transformed into testosterone by Leydig cells in the testes. LH regulates the initial stage of this process. In this mechanism, androstenedione and dehydroepiandrosterone (DHEA) are two crucial intermediates. Androstenedione turns into testosterone thanks to the enzyme 17-beta-hydroxysteroid dehydrogenase. Blood plasma proteins like albumin and sex hormone binding globulin, as well as a large portion of the testosterone present, are bonded to one another. This major source of protein-bound testosterone provides the body with an overabundance of testosterone hormones. Low blood levels of free testosterone cause tissue-level responses in the seminal vesicles, bone, muscle, and prostate gland. By converting testosterone, the enzyme 5-alpha-reductase produces dihydrotestosterone in cells. Both testosterone and dihydrotestosterone can interact with cell receptors and control how proteins are expressed. In the zona reticularis of the adrenal gland, both men and women produce androgens with weak effects. One example of a weak-acting androgen is dehydroepiandrosterone. Despite having a lesser affinity for testosterone receptors, if produced in high amounts, they can be converted to testosterone in the peripheral tissues [32].

3.1 Transport of testosterone

Because it binds to moving plasma proteins, the amount of testosterone that circulates in blood is higher than its solubility in water. Albumin, corticosteroid binding globulin, and 1 acid glycoprotein are low affinity proteins, whereas SHBG, a protein with high affinity but low capacity, is the most important binding protein. The circulating SHBG, a homodimer comprising two 373 amino acid long glycoprotein subunits, readily binds testosterone [33]. It has one highly-affinity steroid binding site, two N-linked and one O-linked glycosylation sites, and three glycosylation sites. The homodimer's two binding sites exhibit cooperative, dynamic binding affinities with subsequent androgen binding [34]. Although genetic variants can change SHBG's capacity to bind testosterone, acquired liver illness has little impact on this feature [35]. It is yet unclear if pregnancy or other long-term illnesses have an impact on it (when circulating levels increase). Humans but not rodents secrete SHBG into the circulation through the liver. Rodent Sertoli cells release testicular androgen-binding protein, or SHBG, into the seminiferous tubules of the testis [36]. Not the least of which is that the placenta may influence the increase in blood SHBG levels during pregnancy. The levels of circulating SHBG, a byproduct of hepatic secretion and a first-pass liver effect of oral medicines, including sex steroids, are significantly influenced by these effects. The levels of circulating SHBG (and consequently total testosterone) are typically increased (androgens, glucocorticoids) or decreased (first pass effects) as a result of producing supraphysiologic hormone concentrations at the liver, such as those caused by oral administration (first pass effects) or by high-dose parenteral androgen injections (estrogens, thyroxine).

Transdermal, depot implants, and parenteral (non-oral) distribution, which essentially maintain physiological circulating hormone concentrations, have no effect on blood SHBG levels [29], whereas endogenous sex steroids and these techniques do. Acute or chronic liver disease, androgen deficit, obesity, diseases that cause protein loss, non-alcoholic fatty liver disease, and, in rare circumstances, hereditary SHBG insufficiency, all have an impact on the level of SHBG in the blood [37, 38]. In a healthy state, SHBG binds 60–70% of the circulating testosterone, leaving 1–2% unbound or linked to lower affinity, high-capacity binding sites for the remainder (albumin, 1 acid glycoprotein, corticosteroid binding protein).

The physicochemical partitioning between the hydrophobic protein binding sites on circulating binding proteins, the hydrophilic aqueous extracellular fluid, and the lipophilic cellular plasma membranes is the basis for the hypothesis that the transport of hydrophobic steroids into tissues occurs passively. The most physiologically active component of testosterone is thought to be the fraction that is weakly protein-bound but still mobile [39], whereas the majority of the moiety that is strongly coupled to SHBG just serves as an inert storage [34].

The free hormone hypothesis is based on the now-outdated pharmacological theory that drug-drug interactions result from the displacement of mutual protein binding. However, in molecular pharmacology, well-established physiological mechanisms like the activation of the drug transporter, the stimulation of the cytochrome P450 enzyme, and other mechanisms unrelated to binding to circulating proteins have long since supplanted this theory. The free fractions may alternatively be viewed of as the least active and transitory since they would have easier access to regions where testosterone is inactivated by degradative metabolism, ultimately stopping androgen action. This would undermine the assumption of the free hormone hypothesis.

So far, it has not been possible to determine the free or bioavailable fractions' overall biological significance. Additionally, evidence from experiments suggests that SHBG actively participates in cellular testosterone uptake through a number of SHBG membrane receptors, uptake processes, and signaling via G protein and cyclic AMP [40]. This is in contrast to the conventional view that SHBG is biologically inert. By facilitating receptor-mediated cellular uptake of SHBG laden with testosterone via endocytosis on cell surface membranes, megalin, a multivalent low-density lipoprotein endocytic receptor, may change tissue androgen activity. Due to its lack of a physiological basis and the scant and speculative empirical data backing it [41], the free hormone hypothesis [42] is thus refuted by broad, prospective clinical inquiry.

Therefore, the biological importance of fractionating circulating testosterone into these derived forms is unknown, and their therapeutic use may be deceptive. The time-consuming, manual techniques necessary for the direct estimation of free testosterone are also only available in research or specialist pathology institutions. They are expensive and lack any external quality control procedures or established reference ranges when they are given.

3.2 Metabolism of testosterone

A very little amount of released testosterone is activated to two bioactive metabolites, estradiol and DHT, by hepatic phase I and II metabolism, whereas the bulk is inactivated to inactive oxidized and conjugated metabolites for urine and/or biliary clearance [43]. The amplification pathway transforms 4% of the blood's testosterone into DHT, a more potent, pure androgen. When transactivating the androgen receptor, DHT has a higher binding affinity and a 3–10 times greater molar potency than testosterone [44]. The most potent natural androgen, DHT, is produced by the 5-reductase enzyme, which is derived from two distinct genes (I and II).

Type 1 5′-reductase is located in the liver, kidney, skin, and brain, whereas type 2 5′-reductase is typically strongly expressed in the prostate but also found in the skin (hair follicles) and liver at smaller levels.

Puberty causes marked virilization, including phallic growth, normal testis development and spermatogenesis, bone density, and, in rare cases, masculine gender reorientation, despite the fact that undermasculinization and congenital 5-reductase deficiency cause genetic males who may be raised as females to experience a specific type of genital ambiguity [1]. While the prostate is still developing, the usual prostate condition is sparse body hair without baldness [45]. The anomalous natural history makes it evident that high levels of 5-reductase expression are necessary as a local androgen amplification mechanism for correct development of the tissues derived from the urogenital sinus. The development of azasteroid 5-reductase inhibitors was based on this mechanism of enhanced androgen activity [46].

Blocking the type 2 5′-reductase enzyme limits the inhibition of testosterone action to the prostate (and other urogenital sinus tissue derivatives) without obstructing extra-prostatic androgen action because it converts over 95% of testosterone entering the prostate into the more potent androgen DHT. However, type 2 5′-reductase mutations result in abnormalities of urogenital sinus derived tissues in both men and mice, whereas genetic inactivation of type 1 5′-reductase has no male phenotype in mice and no mutations of the human type 1 enzyme have been observed [47]. Whether this denotes an unanticipated type 1 enzyme phenotype or a critical role that has persisted throughout evolution, it is unknown.

Through the androgen action diversification pathway, the enzyme aromatase converts testosterone into estradiol to activate estrogen receptors [1]. Although aromatization only contributes 0.2% to testosterone output, because to the increased molar potency of estradiol, it may represent a significant mechanism for diversifying androgen effect in tissues where aromatase is expressed (approximately 100 times higher than testosterone). The diversification route is regulated by the cytochrome P450 enzyme CYP19 aromatase [48]. Extratesticular aromatization is responsible for producing around 80% of the estradiol that is present in eugonadal men.

Beginning in the 1970s, it was shown that the local conversion of testosterone to estradiol inside neural tissues played a key role in mediating testosterone action on the brain, including negative feedback as well as activational and organizational effects [49]. As a result, the biological importance of aromatization in male physiology was acknowledged for the first time [50]. Recent studies have demonstrated the importance of local aromatization in testosterone action by demonstrating that hereditary aromatase inactivation, which results in a complete lack of estrogen, produces substantial developmental abnormalities in the bone and other tissues of men and mice [51]. This illness and genetic changes in mice and men that inactivate ER share a number of commonalities [52]. Additionally, exogenous estrogen or other estrogen-like medicines significantly accelerated bone development in patients with aromatase insufficiency.

Male mice are unaffected by ER genetic inactivation, and no modifications in humans have been seen [53]. The expression of aromatases, which affects local tissue-specific androgen activity via aromatization in tissues like bone [54] and the brain [52], may have an impact on development and function. A mature liver and muscle are two more tissues that exhibit minimal to no aromatase expression. Despite the importance of aromatization in the physiology of male bones, recent research shows that androgens acting through androgen receptors have significant extra direct effects on bone.

Despite having lower levels of circulating estradiol than young women, men have higher bone density than young women [55], non-aromatizable androgens increase bone density in estrogen-deficient women [56], and androgen insensitive rats with non-functional androgen receptors do not maintain normal male bone density [57]. The effects of testosterone on bone and the brain cannot be fully described as a pro-hormone for local estradiol synthesis (and/or action via estrogen receptors and/or). Androgen receptor-mediated actions must be present for testosterone's entire range of effects on the brain and bone to be observed. Regarding the need for aromatization to offset testosterone's effects on male sexual function, conflicting information is available. Male sexual activity was not necessary for aromatization, according to a study that generated estrogen deficiency using DHT and found [58]; however, a different study that produced estrogen deficiency using aromatase inhibitors showed partial dependence.

Therefore, more research is needed to completely understand how aromatization contributes to the maintenance of androgen activity in mature male animals. Notably, testosterone is metabolized to inactive metabolites in the liver, kidney, stomach, muscle, and adipose tissue. Phase I metabolism involves the majority of oxygen moieties being oxidized by hepatic oxidases, particularly those in the cytochrome P450 3A family. Hepatic conjugation to glucuronides during phase II metabolism produces compounds that are sufficiently hydrophilic for renal excretion. The UDP glucuronosyl transferase (UGT) enzymes UGT2B7, UGT2B15, and UGT2B17 catalyze the majority of the phase II metabolism (glucuronidation) of testosterone, with 2B17 being quantitatively the most important. A functional polymorphism of UGT 2B17, a deletion mutation that is several times more common in Asian than European populations, accounts for the concordant population difference in the testosterone to epitestosterone (T/E) ratio in a World AntiDoping Agency-approved urine screening test for testosterone doping in sport, which constitutes an ethnic differential, false negative in surveillance for exogenous testosterone doping [59].

Furthermore, increased blood levels of SHBG, decreased hepatic blood flow (from, for example, posture), or both can slow down the metabolic clearance rate of testosterone. The metabolic inactivation of testosterone could theoretically be impacted by medications that alter hepatic oxidase activity, however there aren't many empirical instances with a big enough effect on clinical practice. The brief duration of action and low oral bioavailability of testosterone when taken parenterally are both brought on by the liver's quick metabolic inactivation. Because of these limitations, oral

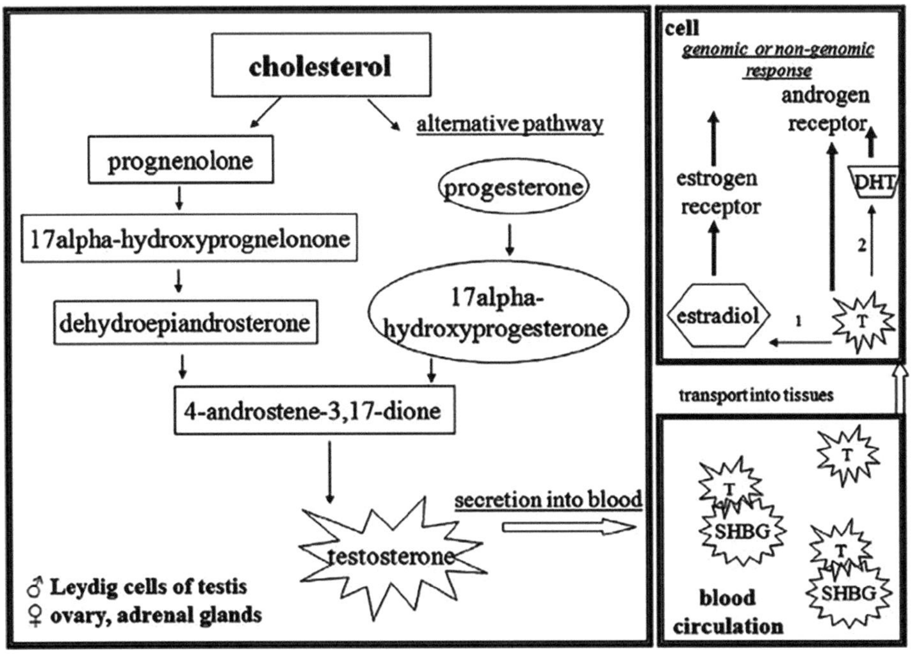

Figure 1.
The metabolism of testosterone. Desmolase activity converts cholesterol into the steroid hormone testosterone [60].

administration methods including buccal, sublingual, and gut lymphatic must either prevent hepatic portal absorption or use synthetic androgens with substituents that prevent them from being inactivated by first pass hepatic metabolism [60] (**Figure 1**).

4. Biological actions of testosterone

The basic sexual processes of spermatogenesis, testicular descent, penis and testes enlargement, and heightened libido are all mediated by testosterone [1]. Around 7 months during the pregnancy, the testes begin to move into the scrotum and begin secreting enough testosterone. Testosterone injections can assist the testes descend via the inguinal canals in male neonates who are born with normal, undescended testes that do not descend by the time they are 4–6 months old. Additionally, testosterone controls the secondary characteristics of males that define their masculinity. Male hair patterns, vocal changes, and voice deepening are examples of secondary sex characteristics in men, in addition to anabolic effects like puberty growth spurts (testosterone increases tissue growth at the epiphyseal plate early on and eventually causes plate closure later in puberty) and skeletal muscle growth (testosterone stimulates protein synthesis) [32]. In addition to increasing erythropoiesis, testosterone causes men to have a greater hematocrit than women. As men age, their testicular size decreases, their libido declines, their muscular mass declines, their production of fat increases, and their erythropoiesis decreases, all of which may contribute to anemia. The biological actions of testosterone could be splitted into two pathway:

4.1 Non-genomic pathway of testosterone

Steroid hormones' non-genomic effects are those steroid-mediated processes that are quick to respond, utilize second messengers, and do not directly involve gene transcription (as seen by their susceptibility to transcriptional and protein synthesis inhibitors) (within seconds to minutes). Non-genomic actions are distinct from genomic mechanisms in that they bind the steroid to an androgen receptor on the cell membrane or establish a connection with a plasma membrane receptor connected to a Pertussis toxin (PTX)-sensitive G protein rather than the more typical androgen receptor found in the cell's cytoplasm before being translocated into the nucleus. In contrast to genomic effects, non-genomic actions of steroid hormones call for the hormone to be present continually. The non-genomic effects will diminish as soon as the hormone leaves the tissue [61–64].

- The most consistent non-genomic consequence of androgen exposure is a fast shift in [Ca2+], despite the fact that the evidence for non-genomic androgen action is sparse. It has been assumed that in order to trigger calcium modulation, which happens within seconds to minutes, the androgen must attach to a receptor on the cell's surface. It's interesting to note that not all cell types that show a rapid androgen Numerous cell types, including osteoblasts, macrophages, T-lymphocytes, endothelial cells, breast cancer cells, prostate cancer cells, androgens' ability to quickly modify the function of ion channels and [Ca2+]i has been noted [61–63].

- Androgens may mediate a range of non-genomic actions through their structural characteristics, independent of receptors, channels, or second messenger pathways. It has been discovered that androgen metabolites can pick up extra charges from sulfate residues, which enables them to enter the lipid/protein complex of the cell membrane and reduce membrane flexibility. This in turn affects how ATP hydrolysis-related enzymes behave [62]. As well as other second messenger pathways, testosterone has been shown to quickly activate calcium pathways. Further proving that androgens are to blame for the downregulation of G activity, testosterone has been shown to decrease potassium input in Xenopus oocytes overexpressing G-protein inward rectifying potassium channels. Interestingly, the effects of T on potassium channel function were prevented by RNA interference-mediated downregulation of AR expression at low but not high T dosages [62].

- Androgens have instantaneous effects on biological systems, as is well documented. The neuroendocrine control of gonadotropin-releasing hormone is one area in particular where androgens and the reproductive system interact intimately (GnRH). It has long been understood that androgens inhibit the anterior pituitary's ability to secrete luteinizing hormone, which is directly controlled by the brain's release of GnRH. Despite the fact that androgens are known to affect the pituitary's sensitivity to GnRH, a new study strongly suggests a neuronal mechanism [1, 32].

- Despite the fact that the specific mechanism of action of androgen treatment is yet unknown, it has been shown that animal behavior changes swiftly in reaction to it. Researchers have shown that utilizing the female lordosis reflex as the end goal, androgens can quickly modify a female rodent's sexual receptivity. Rodents' sexual receptivity is found to be terminated by dihydrotestosterone and 3-Diol, and this effect is shown even when the hormone isn't operating [62].

- Androgens' impact on the central nervous system can be neurotoxic or neuroprotective. It has been determined that dihydrotestosterone can influence cellular development, differentiation, survival, or death through both genomic and non-genomic signaling pathways. When employed in culture, androgens such as T and DHT can protect neurons from damage brought on by beta-amyloid toxicity, kainic acid toxicity, and serum deprivation [62].

- It is clear that testosterone has a negative impact on the cardiovascular system since men are more likely than premenopausal women to have cardiovascular disease. However, numerous clinical and epidemiological studies did find a controversial connection between testosterone and cardiovascular disease. Additionally, an increasing amount of evidence points to the possibility that testosterone may exert its vasorelaxing properties immediately via non-genomic routes. These actions do not require the endothelium, but some studies do indicate an endothelial function. This has a major impact on the vascular smooth muscle [65, 66].

4.2 Genomic pathway of testosterone

The ligand activated receptor is a crucial transcription factor in the genomic route that controls the expression of genes involved in cell division, proliferation, metabolism, and apoptosis. However, the following highlights could be made of testosterone's genomic effects:

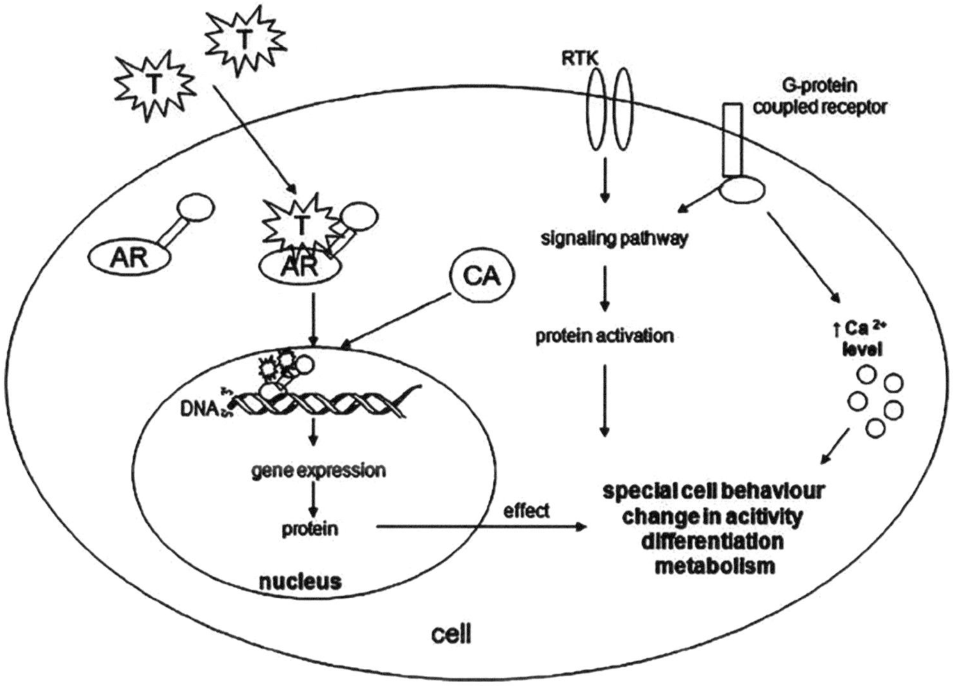

Figure 2.
Depicted the effects of testosterone on both genes and non-genes. Free bioactive testosterone interacts with the cytoplasmic androgen receptor (AR).

- Vascular calcification is the abnormal mineral deposition in the vascular system. Vascular calcification can be controlled. It can occur in the heart's valves and takes on a variety of shapes, such as medial and intimal calcification. Males who had low or high testosterone levels had a higher chance of developing vascular calcification [67].

- Maintaining healthy renal and heart function. A common symptom of Fabry disease, which is brought on by a lack of the lysosomal enzyme—galactosidase A, is cardiac and renal hypertrophy [68].

- Preservation of erectile abilities. It is important to highlight that decreased testosterone expression may, in turn, contribute to the ED vascular phenotype (**Figure 2**) [68].

5. Health benefits of high testosterone

Men with high testosterone levels have been shown to have longer, healthier lives as well as to preserve their sexual potency [69, 70]. Beyond fostering aggression, body and facial hair, and even pattern baldness, testosterone has many other functions as well. Additionally, studies have demonstrated that testosterone protects against autoimmune disease. Since testosterone is an anabolic, it encourages the development of new muscle. One of the main aspects of aging in both men and women is the loss of lean body mass. This loss is made up by testosterone [70]. The most significant study about the link between high levels of testosterone and lowered risk of cardiovascular disease was published in May 1994 and found that low levels of free testosterone are a risk factor and directly correlate with the severity of coronary artery disease.

Lower levels of testosterone have been seen in males with dementia in several studies, which has prompted speculation that testosterone deficiency may contribute to the onset of dementia. However, other research has demonstrated that there is no distinction in testosterone levels between men with dementia and those without it. There is yet no conclusive proof that testosterone levels are correlated with a lower incidence of dementia. Therefore, it is doubtful that using testosterone can help lower your risk of developing dementia. In addition, there are dangers associated with hormone use that must be weighed against your own health.

5.1 Factors that promote and inhibit testosterone secretion

Certain elements can either increase or decrease testosterone levels. Since the building block for male sex hormones is the cholesterol molecule, a low-fat diet restricts the creation of testosterone. Additionally, testosterone is increased by rigorous exercise, but it can be decreased by overtraining [71]. Although severe stress or sadness can suppress testosterone, sexual activity also increases it. While many elderly men can still bear children, their sperm counts may be lower.

5.2 Therapeutics implications of testosterone

Male hypogonadism is mostly treated with androgen replacement therapy, which is the principal application of testosterone. The testosterone injectable preparation called testosterone undecanoate allows for injections every 12 weeks as opposed to every 2–3 weeks as is the case with testosterone esters like testosterone cypionate or enantate. This testosterone injectable preparation also delivers the most consistent blood levels of testosterone, within the physiological range. Short-acting medications lessen the possibility of mood swings or emotional instability by limiting variations in blood concentrations [72]. To administer the hormone, testosterone undecanoate can also be administered orally. Additionally, a patch or gel can be used to apply it transdermally.

Additionally, testosterone is used in the treatment of breast cancer in combination with an aromatase inhibitor to restrict estrogen conversion since it directly inhibits the development of mammary cells via the androgen receptor [73]. Despite the fact that oral administration of testosterone effectively increases absorption, gastrointestinal metabolism and significant first-pass hepatic metabolism make roughly 98% of the hormone inert [74]. When taken with food, testosterone undecanoate molecules are absorbed into chylomicrons, significantly bypassing the liver. The substance then travels through the intestinal lymphatic system and enters the peripheral circulation. However, pills with an oily testosterone composition.

Since low-fat meals have poor testosterone undecanoate absorption, the amount of fat in the meal has an impact [74]. Men who received four intramuscular injections of testosterone undecanoate at intervals of 6 weeks had serum testosterone levels that were consistently at or above the lower physiological limit; the upper physiological limit was only briefly surpassed after the third and fourth doses. The half-life and Cmax of testosterone under prolonged therapy were 70.2 days and 32.0 nmol/l, respectively. To achieve physiological values of serum testosterone in nearly all men, it appears that a 12-week injection interval following initial loading doses of testosterone undecanoate at 0 and 6 weeks is sufficient [72].

6. Pathophysiology of testosterone secretion

Overproduction, underproduction, receptor insensitivity, or poor testosterone metabolism are all examples of pathology connected to testosterone [75]. The more typical and extensively studied testosterone diseases include the ones listed below. The following disorders, such as polycystic ovarian syndrome (PCOS) [76], adrenal virilization/adrenal tumors, ovarian or testicular tumors, Cushing syndrome, and as a result of exogenous steroid use, can cause an overproduction of androgens. It's crucial to grasp the variations between testosterone and dehydroepiandrosterone (DHEA), in order to properly comprehend some of these illnesses. The ovaries, testes, and adrenals all create DHEA, which is a relatively mild androgen. DHEA is a precursor of a number of hormones, including estrogen and testosterone. The adrenal glands only contain DHEA in its sulfated form, or DHEAS. Unusual gonadotropin-releasing hormone (GnRH) secreted during polycystic ovarian syndrome increases LH secretion (PCOS). Women with PCOS who take LH have increased androgen produced by their ovarian theca cells, which results in hirsutism, a masculine escutcheon, acne, and androgenic alopecia. Usually, ovarian and adrenal tumors are accompanied by rapidly worsening androgenic symptoms (hirsutism, virilization). An ovarian tumor is most likely to be to blame when DHEAS is normal and testosterone levels are elevated.

When DHEAS is elevated and testosterone levels are typically normal, an adrenal tumor is most likely the cause. Age, some drugs, chemotherapy, problems with the hypothalamus-pituitary axis, intrinsic hypogonadism, cryptorchidism, orchitis, and genetic illnesses including Klinefelter and Kallmann syndrome can all cause reduced testosterone production [77]. The congenital disorder that results in primary hypogonadism most frequently is Klinefelter syndrome. In Klinefelter, inhibin levels fall and FSH levels rise as a result of seminiferous tubule dysgenesis and Sertoli cell loss. Aromatase is upregulated by FSH, which speeds up the process of turning androgens into estrogens [78]. Because there is no negative feedback when Leydig cells die in Klinefelter, testosterone levels fall and LH levels rise. The Kallmann syndrome, which is characterized by the inability of GnRH-producing neurons to migrate, manifests as a lack of GnRH [78]. LH, FSH, testosterone, and sperm levels fall as a result of low GnRH levels. Compared to other types of hypogonadotropic hypogonadism, Kallmann syndrome is the only one to have defects in the sense of smell (hyposmia or anosmia). Dihydrotestosterone is created from testosterone by an enzyme known as 5-alpha reductase [65]. Due to a shortage of dihydrotestosterone, males with 5-alpha reductase insufficiency may be born with ambiguous genitalia or with typical female or male genitalia. The internal male urogenital tract is present in these folks (anti-Mullerian hormone is still present). Teenagers with this enzyme deficit, who may have been raised as girls due to a lack of secondary male characteristics, begin to develop secondary male sex characteristics and experience primary amenorrhea at puberty [79]. Less DHT and a higher testosterone to DHT ratio will be present in these people, who will also have normal levels of LH and testosterone.

Patients with androgen insensitivity, as opposed to those with insufficient levels of the enzyme 5-alpha reductase, are less virilized due to the absence of functional androgen receptors. Similar to those who have a 5-alpha reductase impairment, these patients exhibit a 46 XY karyotype [66]. On the other hand, these patients have typical undescended testes and healthy external genitalia. During adolescence, they experience primary amenorrhea and the development of their breasts, but not the vocal changes or pubic or axillary hair growth associated with puberty. They will have a defective internal reproductive system and a blind vaginal pouch as a result of the Mullerian inhibitory factor being created. These people will have very high levels of LH and testosterone. Several types of congenital adrenal hyperplasia (CAH) may have impaired testosterone metabolism as a secondary consequence [80]. In 95% of instances with typical CAH, which is caused by a lack of 21 hydroxylase, neonates first display ambiguous genitalia. Later, they experience vomiting, hypotension, acidosis, salt deficiency, and other symptoms. Hyperandrogenism results from a significant increase in 17-hydroxyprogesterone being diverted to adrenal androgen production. By dramatically raising GnRH production, which boosts LH and FSH levels, hyperandrogenism decreases the hypothalamic sensitivity to progesterone. The generation of gonadal steroids increases when LH and FSH levels rise (17-hydroxyprogesterone, DHEA, testosterone, LH, and FSH). The diagnosis is made by the adrenocorticotropic hormone stimulation test, which displays an excessive 17-hydroxyprogesterone response.

7. Concluding remarks

Both men and women produce testosterone, which is one of the most significant sex hormones. Leydig cells from men's testicles create the majority of it. In males, the adrenal cortex also releases it. The development of secondary sexual traits in males, such as increased muscle, bone mass, and body and facial hair, is widely acknowledged to be heavily influenced by testosterone. Maintaining sexual potency, on the other hand, is critical. Furthermore, testosterone has been found in studies to protect against autoimmune disorders.

Author details

Oyovwi Mega Obukohwo[1*], Ben-Azu Benneth[2], Ovuakporaye Irikefe Simon[3], Onome Bright Oghenetega[4], Emojevwe Victor[5], Falajiki Y. Faith[1], Patrick Godwin Okwute[4], Rotu Arientare Rume[6], Okoro Ogheneyebrorue Godswill[7] and Nwangwa Eze Kingsley[3]

1 Department of Physiology, Adeleke University, Ede, Osun State, Nigeria

2 Faculty of Basic Medical Science, Department of Pharmacology, College of Health Sciences, Delta State University, Abraka, Delta State, Nigeria

3 Faculty of Basic Medical Health Science, Department of Physiology, Delta State University, Nigeria

4 Department of Physiology, School of Basic Medical Science, Babcock University, Illisan, Nigeria

5 Department of Physiology, University of Medical Sciences, Ondo, Ondo State, Nigeria

6 Department of Physiology, University of Ibadan, Ibadan, Oyo State, Nigeria

7 Department of Anatomy, Achievers University, Owo, Ondo State, Nigeria

*Address all correspondence to: megalect@gmail.com

References

[1] Oyovwi Mega Obukohwo, Nwangwa Eze Kingsley, Rotu Arientare Rume and Emojevwe Victor (2022): The concept of male reproductive anatomy. 3-34. (Male Reproductive Anatomy by Wu, W., (Ed.). (2022). London, UK IntechOpen. DOI:10.5772/intechopen.94696

[2] Freeman ER, Bloom DA, McGuire EJ. A brief history of testosterone. The Journal of Urology. 2001;**165**(2):371-373

[3] David K, Dingemanse E, Freud J, Laqueur E. Über krystallinisches männliches Hormon aus Hoden (Testosteron), wirksamer als aus Harn oder aus Cholesterin bereitetes Androsteron. 1935:281-283

[4] Kenyon AT. The effect of testosterone propionate on the genitalia, prostate, secondary sex characters, and body weight in eunuchoidism. Endocrinology. 1938;**23**(2):121-134

[5] Møller J, Einfeldt H. Historical review. In: Testosterone Treatment of Cardiovascular Diseases. Berlin, Heidelberg: Springer; 1984. pp. 1-3

[6] Waldman S. The treatment of angina pectoris with testosterone propionate. The Journal of Clinical Endocrinology. 1945;**5**(7):305-317

[7] Hamwi GJ. Marfan's syndrome (arachnodactyly). The American Journal of Medicine. 1951;**11**(2):261-266

[8] Hartgens F, Kuipers H. Effects of androgenic-anabolic steroids in athletes. Sports Medicine. 2004;**34**(8):513-554

[9] Katz AM, Katz PB. Diseases of heart in works of Hippocrates. British Heart Journal. 1962;**24**:257-264

[10] Lawrence JH, Tobias CA, Linfoot JA, Born JL, Gottschalk A, Kling RP. Heavy particles, the Bragg curve and suppression of pituitary function in diabetic retinopathy. Diabetes. 1963;**12**(6):490-501

[11] Kim SH, Park JJ, Kim KH, Yang HJ, Kim DS, Lee CH, et al. Efficacy of testosterone replacement therapy for treating metabolic disturbances in late-onset hypogonadism: A systematic review and meta-analysis. International Urology and Nephrology. 2021;**53**(9):1733-1746

[12] Phillips GB, Pinkernell BH, Jing T-Y. The association of hypotestosteronemia with coronary artery disease in men. Arherosclerosis and Thrombosis. 1994;**14**(5):701-706

[13] Miller WL, Auchus RJ. The molecular biology, biochemistry, and physiology of human steroidogenesis and its disorders. Endocrine Reviews. 2011;**32**:81-151

[14] Peng HM, Im SC, Pearl NM, Turcu AF, Rege J, Waskell L, et al. Cytochrome b5 activates the 17,20-lyase activity of human cytochrome P450 17A1 by increasing the coupling of NADPH consumption to androgen production. Biochemistry. 2016;**55**:4356-4365

[15] Davison SL, Bell R, Donath S, Montalto JG, Davis SR. Androgen levels in adult females: Changes with age, menopause, and oophorectomy. Journal of Clinical Endocrinology and Metabolism. 2005;**90**:3847-3853

[16] Labrie F. Adrenal androgens and intracrinology. Seminars in Reproductive Medicine. 2004;**22**:299-309

[17] Gallegos AM, Atshaves BP, Storey SM, Starodub O, Petrescu AD, Huang H, et al. Gene structure, intracellular localization,

and functional roles of sterol carrier protein-2. Progress in Lipid Research. 2001;**40**:498-563

[18] Miller WL. Disorders in the initial steps of steroid hormone synthesis. The Journal of Steroid Biochemistry and Molecular Biology. 1 Jan 2017;**165**:18-37

[19] Midzak A, Zirkin B, Papadopoulos V. Translocator protein: Pharmacology and steroidogenesis. Biochemical Society Transactions. 2015;**43**:572-578

[20] Jarow JP, Zirkin BR. The androgen microenvironment of the human testis and hormonal control of spermatogenesis. Annals of the New York Academy of Sciences. 2005;**1061**:208-220

[21] Kaufman JM, Vermeulen A. The decline of androgen levels in elderly men and its clinical and therapeutic implications. Endocrine Reviews. 2005;**26**:833-876

[22] Sartorius G, Spasevska S, Idan A, Turner L, Forbes E, Zamojska A, et al. Serum testosterone, dihydrotestosterone and estradiol concentrations in older men self-reporting very good health: The healthy man study. Clinical Endocrinology. 2012;**77**:755-763

[23] Feldman HA, Longcope C, Derby CA, Johannes CB, Araujo AB, Coviello AD, et al. Age trends in the level of serum testosterone and other hormones in middle-aged men: Longitudinal results from the Massachusetts male aging study. Journal of Clinical Endocrinology and Metabolism. 2002;**87**:589-598

[24] Perheentupa A, Makinen J, Laatikainen T, Vierula M, Skakkebaek NE, Andersson AM, et al. A cohort effect on serum testosterone levels in Finnish men. European Journal of Endocrinology. 2013;**168**:227-233

[25] Sikaris K, McLachlan RI, Kazlauskas R, de Kretser D, Holden CA, Handelsman DJ. Reproductive hormone reference intervals for healthy fertile young men: Evaluation of automated platform assays. Journal of Clinical Endocrinology and Metabolism. 2005;**90**:5928-5936

[26] Veldhuis JD, Keenan DM, Liu PY, Iranmanesh A, Takahashi PY, Nehra AX. The aging male hypothalamic-pituitary-gonadal axis: Pulsatility and feedback. Molecular and Cellular Endocrinology. 2009;**299**:14-22

[27] Nair KS, Rizza RA, O'Brien P, Dhatariya K, Short KR, Nehra A, et al. DHEA in elderly women and DHEA or testosterone in elderly men. New England Journal of Medicine. 2006;**355**:1647-1659

[28] Santner S, Albertson B, Zhang GY, Zhang GH, Santulli M, Wang C, et al. Comparative rates of androgen production and metabolism in Caucasian and Chinese subjects. Journal of Clinical Endocrinology and Metabolism. 1998;**83**:2104-2109

[29] Wang C, Cunningham G, Dobs A, Iranmanesh A, Matsumoto AM, Snyder PJ, et al. Long-term testosterone gel (AndroGel) treatment maintains beneficial effects on sexual function and mood, lean and fat mass, and bone mineral density in hypogonadal men. Journal of Clinical Endocrinology and Metabolism. 2004;**89**:2085-2098

[30] Diver MJ, Imtiaz KE, Ahmad AM, Vora JP, Fraser WD. Diurnal rhythms of serum total, free and bioavailable testosterone and of SHBG in middle-aged men compared with those in young men. Clinical Endocrinology. 2003;**58**:710-717

[31] Jin G, Sun J, Kim ST, Feng J, Wang Z, Tao S, et al. Genome-wide association study identifies a new locus JMJD1C

at 10q21 that may influence serum androgen levels in men. Human Molecular Genetics. 2012;**21**:5222-5228

[32] Victor E, Osarugue I, Obukohwo OM, Kingsley NE, Obidike NA. Endocrine Functions of the Testes. In: Male Reproductive Anatomy. IntechOpen; 11 Nov 2021

[33] Hammond GL, Wu TS, Simard M. Evolving utility of sex hormone-binding globulin measurements in clinical medicine. Current Opinion in Endocrinology, Diabetes, and Obesity. 2012;**19**:183-189

[34] Goldman AL, Bhasin S, Wu FCW, Krishna M, Matsumoto AM, Jasuja R. A reappraisal of testosterone's binding in circulation: Physiological and clinical implications. Endocrine Reviews. 2017;**38**:302-324

[35] Wu TS, Hammond GL. Naturally occurring mutants inform SHBG structure and function. Molecular Endocrinology. 2014;**28**:1026-1038

[36] Selva DM, Hammond GL. Human sex hormone-binding globulin is expressed in testicular germ cells and not in sertoli cells. Hormone and Metabolic Research. 2006;**38**:230-235

[37] Sarkar M, VanWagner LB, Terry JG, Carr JJ, Rinella M, Schreiner PJ, et al. Sex hormone-binding globulin levels in young men are associated with nonalcoholic fatty liver disease in midlife. The American Journal of Gastroenterology. 2019;**114**:758-763

[38] Vos MJ, Mijnhout GS, Rondeel JM, Baron W, Groeneveld PH. Sex hormone binding globulin deficiency due to a homozygous missense mutation. Journal of Clinical Endocrinology and Metabolism. 2014;**99**:E1798-E1802

[39] Ekins R. Measurement of free hormones in blood. Endocrine Reviews. 1990;**11**:5-46

[40] Hamada A, Sissung T, Price DK, Danesi R, Chau CH, Sharifi N, et al. Effect of SLCO1B3 haplotype on testosterone transport and clinical outcome in caucasian patients with androgen-independent prostatic cancer. Clinical Cancer Research. 2008;**14**:3312-3318

[41] Hsu B, Cumming RG, Blyth FM, Naganathan V, Waite LM, Le Couteur DG, et al. Evaluating calculated free testosterone as a predictor of morbidity and mortality independent of testosterone for cross-sectional and 5-year longitudinal health outcomes in older men: The Concord Health and Ageing in Men Project. The Journals of Gerontology. Series A, Biological Sciences and Medical Sciences. 2018;**73**:729-736

[42] Handelsman DJ. Free testosterone: Pumping up the tires or ending the free ride? Endocrine Reviews. 2017;**38**:297-301

[43] Van Eenoo P, Delbeke FT. Metabolism and excretion of anabolic steroids in doping control—New steroids and new insights. Journal of Steroid Biochemistry and Molecular Biology. 2006;**101**:161-178

[44] McRobb L, Handelsman DJ, Kazlauskas R, Wilkinson S, McLeod MD, Heather AK. Structure-activity relationships of synthetic progestins in a yeast-based in vitro androgen bioassay. Journal of Steroid Biochemistry and Molecular Biology. 2008;**110**:39-47

[45] Imperato-McGinley J, Zhu YS. Androgens and male physiology the syndrome of 5alpha-reductase-2

deficiency. Molecular and Cellular Endocrinology. 2002;**198**:51-59

[46] Steers WD. 5alpha-reductase activity in the prostate. Urology. 2001;**58**:17-24

[47] Zhu YS, Katz MD, Imperato-McGinley J. Natural potent androgens: Lessons from human genetic models. Baillieres Clinical Endocrinology and Metabolism. 1998;**12**:83-113

[48] Bulun SE, Takayama K, Suzuki T, Sasano H, Yilmaz B, Sebastian S. Organization of the human aromatase p450 (CYP19) gene. Seminars in Reproductive Medicine. 2004;**22**:5-9

[49] Naftolin F. Brain aromatization of androgens. Journal of Reproductive Medicine. 1994;**39**:257-261

[50] Roselli CF. Brain aromatase: Roles in reproduction and neuroprotection. Journal of Steroid Biochemistry and Molecular Biology. 2007;**106**:143-150

[51] Jones ME, Boon WC, Proietto J, Simpson ER. Of mice and men: The evolving phenotype of aromatase deficiency. Trends in Endocrinology and Metabolism. 2006;**17**:55-64

[52] Lubahn DB, Moyer JS, Golding TS, Couse JF, Korach KS, Smithies O. Alteration of reproductive function but not prenatal sexual development after insertional disruption of the mouse estrogen receptor gene. Proceedings of the National Academy of Sciences USA. 1993;**90**:11162-11166

[53] Couse JE, Mahato D, Eddy EM, Korach KS. Molecular mechanism of estrogen action in the male: Insights from the estrogen receptor null mice. Reproduction, Fertility, and Development. 2001;**13**:211-219

[54] Gennari L, Nuti R, Bilezikian JP. Aromatase activity and bone homeostasis in men. Journal of Clinical Endocrinology and Metabolism. 2004;**89**:5898-5907

[55] Vanderschueren D, Vandenput L, Boonen S, Lindberg MK, Bouillon R, Ohlsson C. Androgens and bone. Endocrine Reviews. 2004;**25**:389-425

[56] Need AG, Nordin BEC, Chatterton BE. Double-blind placebo-controlled trial of treatment of osteoporosis with the anabolic steroid nandrolone decanoate. Osteoporosis International. 1993;**3**(Suppl. 1):S218-S222

[57] Vandenput L, Swinnen JV, Boonen S, Van Herck E, Erben RG, Bouillon R, et al. Role of the androgen receptor in skeletal homeostasis: The androgen-resistant testicular feminized male mouse model. Journal of Bone and Mineral Research. 2004;**19**:1462-1470

[58] Sartorius GA, Ly LP, Handelsman DJ. Male sexual function can be maintained without aromatization: Randomized placebo-controlled trial of dihydrotestosterone (DHT) in healthy, older men for 24 months. The Journal of Sexual Medicine. 2014;**11**:2562-2570

[59] Jakobsson J, Ekstrom L, Inotsume N, Garle M, Lorentzon M, Ohlsson C, et al. Large differences in testosterone excretion in Korean and Swedish men are strongly associated with a UDP-glucuronosyl transferase 2B17 polymorphism. Journal of Clinical Endocrinology and Metabolism. 2006;**91**:687-693

[60] Kurz D. Current management of undescended testes. Current Treatment Options in Pediatrics. 2016;**2**(1):43-51. DOI: 10.1007/s40746-016-0039-7 Epub 2016 Jan 25. PMID: 27158583; PMCID: PMC4856300

[61] Perusquía M. Androgens and non-genomic vascular responses in hypertension. Biochemical Pharmacology. 1 Aug 2022:115200

[62] Foradori CD, Weiser MJ, Handa RJ. Non-genomic actions of androgens. Frontiers in Neuroendocrinology. 2008;**29**(2):169-181

[63] Lorigo M, Mariana M, Lemos MC, Cairrao E. Vascular mechanisms of testosterone: The non-genomic point of view. The Journal of Steroid Biochemistry and Molecular Biology. 2020;**196**:105496

[64] Dent JR, Fletcher DK, McGuigan MR. Evidence for a non-genomic action of testosterone in skeletal muscle which may improve athletic performance: Implications for the female athlete. Journal of Sports Science and Medicine. 2012;**11**(3):363

[65] Bozzola M, Bozzola E, Montalbano C, Stamati FA, Ferrara P, Villani A. Delayed puberty versus hypogonadism: A challenge for the pediatrician. Annals of Pediatric Endocrinology & Metabolism. 2018;**23**(2):57-61

[66] Zhang JR, Zhang PY, Sun LG. Mild androgen insensitivity syndrome: A case report. Zhonghua Nei Ke Za Zhi. 2018;**57**(8):600-602

[67] Woodward HJ, Zhu D, Hadoke PW, MacRae VE. Regulatory role of sex hormones in cardiovascular calcification. International Journal of Molecular Sciences. 2021;**22**(9):4620

[68] Lucas-Herald AK, Alves-Lopes R, Montezano AC, Ahmed SF, Touyz RM. Genomic and non-genomic effects of androgens in the cardiovascular system: Clinical implications. Clinical Science. 2017;**131**(13):1405-1418

[69] Rajfer J. Relationship between testosterone and erectile dysfunction. Reviews in Urology. 2000;**2**(2):122

[70] Cunningham GR, Stephens-Shields AJ, Rosen RC, Wang C, Bhasin S, Matsumoto AM, et al. Testosterone treatment and sexual function in older men with low testosterone levels. The Journal of Clinical Endocrinology & Metabolism. 2016;**101**(8):3096-3104

[71] Kraemer RR, Durand RJ, Acevedo EO, Johnson LG, Synovitz LB, Kraemer GR, et al. Effects of high-intensity exercise on leptin and testosterone concentrations in well-trained males. Endocrine. 2003;**21**(3):261-265

[72] Yassin AA, Haffejee M. Testosterone depot injection in male hypogonadism: A critical appraisal. Clinical Interventions in Aging. 2007;**2**(4):577-579

[73] Glaser RL, York AE, Dimitrakakis C. Subcutaneous testosterone-letrozole therapy before and concurrent with neoadjuvant breast chemotherapy: Clinical response andtherapeutic implications. Menopause. 2017;**24**(7):859-864

[74] Schnabel PG, Bagchus W, Lass H, Thomsen T, Geurts TB. The effect of food composition on serum testosterone levels after oral administration of Andriol Testocaps. Clinical Endocrinology (Oxford). 2007;**66**(4):579-585

[75] Nassar GN, Leslie SW. Physiology, testosterone. [Updated 2022 Jan 4]. In: StatPearls [Internet]. Treasure Island (FL): StatPearls Publishing; 2022 Available from: https://www.ncbi.nlm.nih.gov/books/NBK526128/

[76] Walters KA, Bertoldo MJ, Handelsman DJ. Evidence from animal models on the pathogenesis of PCOS.

Best Practice & Research. Clinical Endocrinology & Metabolism. 2018;**32**(3):271-281

[77] Kalfa N, Gaspari L, Ollivier M, Philibert P, Bergougnoux A, Paris F, et al. Molecular genetics of hypospadias and cryptorchidism recent developments. Clinical Genetics. 2019;**95**(1):122-131

[78] Spaziani M, Mileno B, Rossi F, Granato S, Tahani N, Anzuini A, et al. Endocrine and metabolic evaluation of classic Klinefelter syndrome and high-grade aneuploidies of sexual chromosomes with male phenotype: Are they different clinical conditions? European Journal of Endocrinology. 2018;**178**(4):343-352 [PubMed]

[79] Hauser LJ, Jensen EL, Mirsky DM, Chan KH. Pediatric anosmia: A case series. International Journal of Pediatric Otorhinolaryngology. 2018;**110**:135-139

[80] Falhammar H, Filipsson Nyström H, Wedell A, Thoren M. Cardiovascular risk, metabolic profile, and body composition in adult males with congenital adrenal hyperplasia due to 21-hydroxylase deficiency. European Journal of Endocrinology. 2011;**164**(2):285

Section 2

Functions and Uses of Testosterone

Chapter 3

Testosterone Misuse

Zied Kaabia

Abstract

Testosterone is a key compound of the anabolic androgenic steroids (AAS) family. It has largely been misused in human and animal doping targeting a muscle tissue growth and an enhancement of performances. Such practices constitute a violation against ethical values, food safety, and animal welfare. Consequently, the use of such substance is regulated by WADA and International committees for some animal species such as equine and bovine. Although efficient, the detection of testosterone misuse remains challenging in some cases due to its endogenous origin and its inter- and intra-individual level fluctuation in biological fluids. Novel analytical strategies have been developed and are continuously evolving in order to tackle this issue and to provide a better control of testosterone misuse.

Keywords: anti-doping control, analytical chemistry, mass spectrometry, regulation, anabolic androgenic steroids

1. Introduction

"Doping" as a term has usually been correlated to fraudulent practices undertaken by dishonest athletes to improve their sporting results. However, the use of this term overpasses the boundaries of human sport field to cover the field of sports and food-producing animals such as horses and bovine. Androgenic anabolic steroids (AAS) misuse, in particular, represents one of the hottest and most challenging topics in this context.

Testosterone belongs to androgenic anabolic steroids (AAS) family, which is a group of derivatives originating from the cholesterol biosynthesis in mammals or issued from synthetic chemical reactions. These compounds are reported to be masculinizing agents (androgenic) and promoting skeletal muscle building (anabolic) [1, 2]. The interesting anabolic properties were demonstrated for the first time by Brown-Sequard [3], who reported an improvement in strength and force upon an injection of an extract of dog and guinea pig testicles. Based on its beneficial effects, testosterone has originally been used as therapeutical agent for clinical treatments such as the treatment of hypogonadism or anemia. Consequently, the availability of testosterone increased, and its use was diverted from their original purpose.

In addition to their unethical use to enhance performances and produce higher volume of muscle carcasses, these doping practices pop out as a major concern and a threat for human and animal health and welfare.

In food-producing animals, testosterone is often used by unscrupulous cattle breeders in order to stimulate bovine muscle growth and make a higher profit with regard to the consequent gain in weight over a short period of time [4]. The worldwide debate about the use of such practices has existed since the discovery of their misuse. Several international projects such as the "Transatlantic Trade and Investment Partnership" tend to harmonize the laws regarding the use of AAS in the world. These projects are mainly bringing together for negotiating process the European Union countries, which are imposing a strict regulation system regarding the AAS misuse and the USA, regulations of which offer some permissions for the use of some AAS such as estradiol and stanozolol.

The strict regulation toward AAS misuse in food-producing animals adopted by the European Union countries originates from the various scandals that stroke the region due to the misuse of these substances. One of the biggest high-profile scandals occurred in the 1980s in Italy with the discovery of diethylstilbestrol, a growth hormone promoter, in baby food. Consequently, several measures have been taken by the European Union [5, 6]. According to these directives, adequate analytical methods had to be developed and implemented in the different accredited control laboratories in order to guarantee the consumer's security toward these active chemicals [7]. The analytical methods are mainly based on chromatography coupled to mass spectrometry techniques permitting the detection of residues in biological matrices. The system revealed to be efficient for detecting a large spectrum of anabolic strategies. However, some particular cases remain challenging with regard to the current methodologies adopted by reference laboratories. The use of "hormone cocktails" is among these particular issues [8] and consists of the administration of different anabolic agents such as testosterone, each occurring at low concentration levels. These low quantities of anabolic agents cannot be detected with regard to the detectability limitations of the analytical methods. The use of "Designer Drugs" constitutes another issue for control laboratories. Indeed, "Designers" are exclusively xenobiotic substances not listed among prohibited substances. Considering the lack of knowledge on their exact chemical structure, they cannot be detected by the classical targeted analytical strategies. Finally, the use of natural steroids such as testosterone constitutes a challenge for control laboratories with regard to the similar structures exhibited by these administered substances and their corresponding endogenous analogs.

In the equestrian world, "doping" has been in existence since the ancient Roman era where horses were fed with a "magic potion" called "Hydromel," a mixture of milk and honey, in order to improve their physical performances in the Arena. In the twentieth century, administering alkaloids such as cocaine or strytchine to horses emerged as a new doping treatment permitting to minimize the feeling of physical tiredness. The fraudulent use of these exciting substances increased simultaneously with the appearance of horserace bets, which generated important financial gains. In addition, the use of AAS spread considering their power to enhance physical performances. In order to tackle this issue threatening the equestrian world as a whole in terms of ethical values and animal welfare and with the hope to avoid a tarnished image of horse racing competitions, the International Federation of Horseracing Authorities (IFHA) put into practice a strict control system similar to the one regulating athletes doping implemented by the World Anti-Doping Agency (WADA). This control system, "the racing code," forbids the use of any medication during horseracing competitions and bans in particular the use of AAS in horses during training sessions, pre-competition or competition periods. Targeting an efficient application of this control system, IFHA reference laboratories are committed to developing analytical methods mainly based on chromatography coupled to mass spectrometry techniques allowing the identification and quantification of residues in biological matrices. Although being highly efficient, these methods highlighted, similarly to the official analytical methods adopted in food-producing animal field, some limitations for detecting naturally occurring steroids misuse.

2. Structure and pharmacology of steroid hormones

Anabolic-androgenic steroid hormones share the same substructure based on a sterane nucleus (**Figure 1**). The different families of steroid hormones result from the existence of minor modifications occurring at the sterane nucleus. Progestagens such as progesterone, corticosteroids such as cortisone and aldosterone, estrogens such as estradiol, and androgens such as testosterone are some example of these families.

All of these steroids are derived from cholesterol, which is mainly biosynthesized after dietary intake. This steroid biosynthetic pathway begins with an oxidation of the side chain of the cholesterol to form the androgens prior to the formation of estrogens. This oxidation reaction, catalyzed by the Cytochrome P450, generates pregnenolone, which whether can be biotransformed into progesterone through the enzyme 3β-HSD initiating the creation of the progestagen family or into 17α-hydroxypregnenolone through an oxidation by $CP_{17\alpha}$. The latter compound is subsequently metabolized into DHEA and then to 4-androstenedione, precursor of testosterone.

Estrogens are formed during the reaction of aromatization occurring under the action of CP450. The aromatization consists of the oxidation of the methyl group at position C19 and the consecutive elimination of this newly formed to form estrogens such as estrone and estradiol. This reaction results in the creation of secondary products such as nandrolone. All these transformations are summarized in **Figure 2**.

The secretion of naturally occurring hormones is enhanced by the Luteinizing Hormone (LH), which activates the biotransformation of cholesterol into pregnenolone and the Follicle-Stimulating Hormone (FSH), which participates in the aromatization of testosterone into estradiols. The secretion of two latter hormones is regulated by the Gonadotropin-Releasing Hormone (GnRH) according to the occurring plasmatic concentration levels of steroid hormones.

The steroid hormones are subsequently submitted to phase I biotransformations (oxidations, reductions, epimerizations, etc.) and phase II biostransformations (mainly sulfo and glucuruno conjugation) in order to be eliminated predominantly through urine.

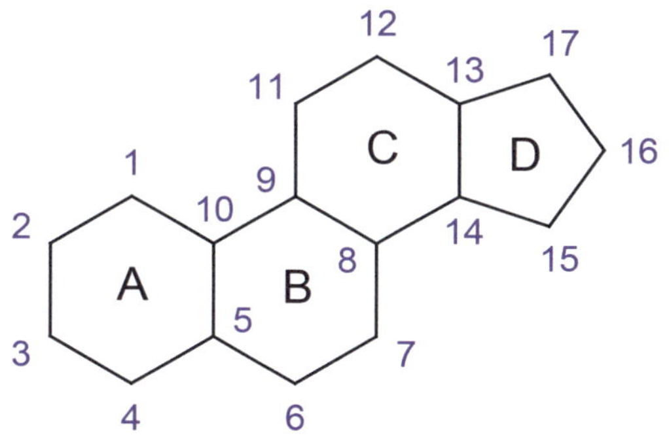

Figure 1.
Structure of a cyclopentanoperhydrophenantrene nucleus or sterane.

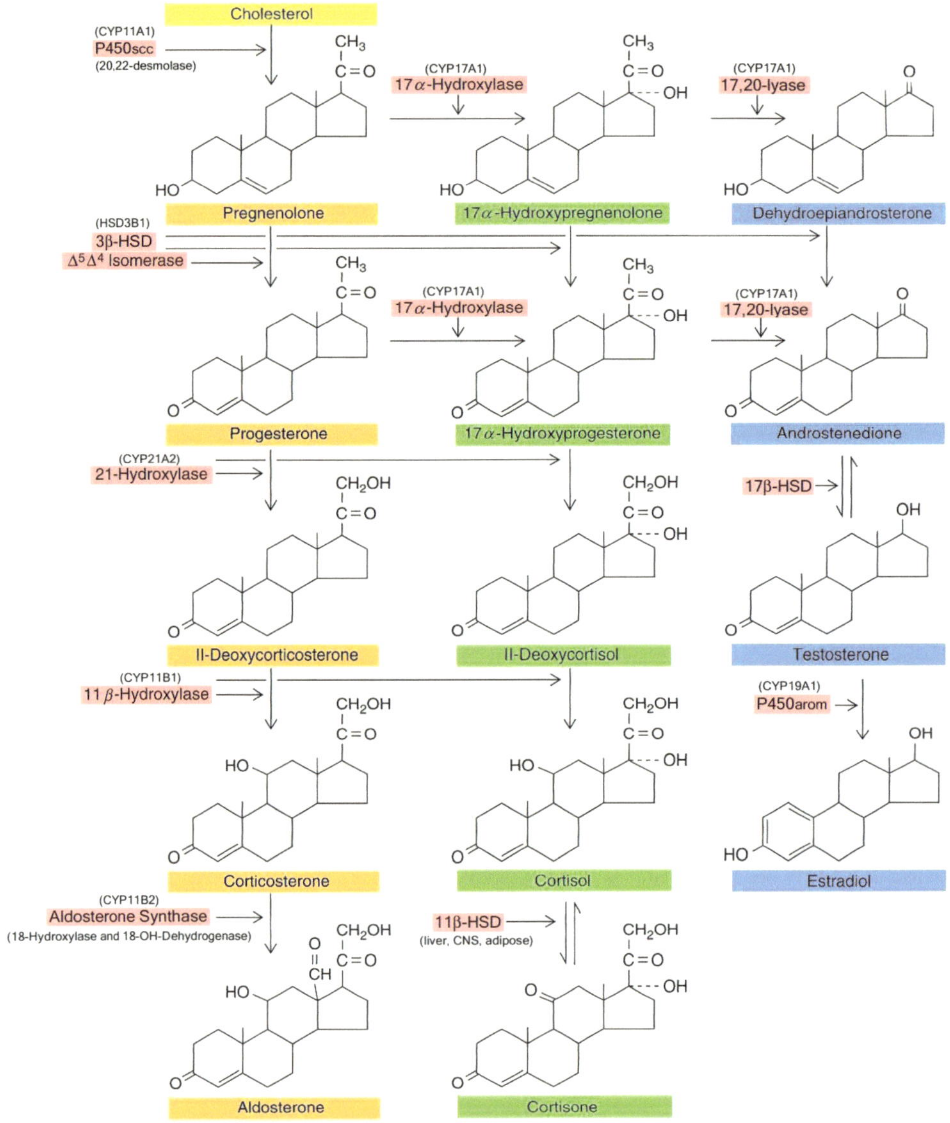

Figure 2.
Global overview of the metabolization products deriving from cholesterol and the occurring biotransformations generating the different steroid families.

The nature of these biotransformations is essentially correlated to the steroid nature and the occurring enzymatic system in the organism. Therefore, the steroids biotransformations present some differences depending on the species. For instance, phase II steroid biotransformations consist mainly of sulfoconjugation reactions in equine species while they consist of glucurunoconjugation reactions in humans and bovine species.

While the previously described steroid hormones such as testosterone occur naturally in the organism, some other steroids are exclusively synthetic. They usually exhibit minor modifications to their endogenous analogues such as methyltestosterone. They can also be part of a new category of steroids called "Designers."

These steroids are unmarketed compounds exhibiting a chemical structure based on marketed substances presenting minor modifications. They are usually synthesized as part of the pharmaceutical industry for medical use. With regard to their inexistence in the list of WADA banned substances, their detection using classical targeted analytical methods becomes problematic. Estra-4,9-diene-3,17-dione [9] and tetrahydrogestrinone [10] are some examples of this category of synthetic compounds.

3. Use of steroid hormones

The use of anabolic steroids in food-producing and sport animals has been flourishing with regard to their capacity to increase zootechnic performances [11, 12]. Testosterone has been one of the main steroids used in this context. Typical quantities of administered steroids to human, bovine, and equine for doping purposes range between hundreds of micrograms and few milligrams per kilogram. The administration of these steroids may be performed orally, through parenteral or alternative pathways:

Oral pathway: minor chemical modifications to the structure of natural anabolic steroids have to be performed prior to an oral administration. These modifications protect the steroid from a submission to a quick metabolization through the hepatic pathway. These modifications consist mainly of an alkylation or an esterification. One example of such steroids is the methyl testosterone, efficiency of which is four times higher than testosterone when administered orally.

Parenteral pathway: this relates to any administration occurring on a different way than the digestive one. When the steroid is administered under its free form through this pathway, it undergoes a quick metabolization leading to its degradation and elimination. Therefore, a step of esterification of the steroid is necessary to provide the desired effect on an extended period of time. The intramuscular administration of the steroid ester is immediately followed by an enzymatic hydrolysis in blood [13]. Prior to hydrolysis, the steroid ester migrates gradually from its lipophilic excipient toward blood stream [14]. This gradual liberation results in a longer effect of the doping substance. The effect is even longer when the steroid ester presents a longer lipophilic side chain [15]. Once the active steroid is formed, it is transferred through the blood stream to the corresponding hormonal receptor.

The administration of the anabolic steroid could be also performed through an intravenous pathway or through solid implants.

Alternative pathways: the transdermal application of steroids is also a possible way for administration with regard to the lipophilic nature of the skin. Anabolic steroids are usually administered through the application of spray or "pour-on" [16]. These pathways have the advantage not to submit the steroids to the first hepatic transition caused by the liver. However, a frequent application is necessary with regard to the low biodisponibility of the steroids using this pathway.

3.1 Transport of steroid hormones

Hormone steroids are rarely present in the blood under their free form. Instead, they are carried in the bloodstream bound to serum carrier proteins [17]. There are two categories of binding proteins:

Non-specific binding carrier proteins: albumin is one example of these binding proteins, and it is characterized by a high capacity of transport but a low affinity with steroids. It is found at a relatively high concentration in blood. Its main function is to ensure the transport of steroids to their corresponding hormonal receptors.

Specific binding carrier proteins: SHBG (Sex Hormones Binding Globulin) is an example of this class of proteins [18]. They are characterized by a high affinity with steroids but a low capacity of transport.

The bioavailability of the endogenous steroids is ensured by these proteins. These proteins play indeed the role of a reservoir of steroids regulating the concentration levels of steroid hormones in the metabolism. Moreover, these proteins protect the transported steroids by preventing their biotransformation and subsequent diffusion and elimination [19].

3.2 Protein production activation

When the steroids reach the target cell, they penetrate through the phospholipidic membrane of the cell by passive diffusion. This passage is guaranteed with regard to the fat-soluble nature of the hormonal steroids. Once inside the cell, the steroids bind to their specific androgenic receptor located in cytoplasm [20]. This binding results in the formation of a steroid-receptor complex, which infiltrates the nucleus to bind to a specific receptor located on chromatine. Consequently, the production of RNA messenger (mRNA) is initiated [21]. These mRNAs are then transported to the cytoplasm for further proteins synthesis.

3.3 Biological effects

The AAS are well-known to enhance muscle growth (anabolic effect) and to promote masculinization (androgenic effect). In addition, the use of these substances may lead to harmful effects such as hypogonadism and cardiovascular risks [22]. These effects are mainly caused by the disturbance occurring through the administration of exogenous steroids, which results in a negative feedback on the secretion of natural steroid hormones. Furthermore, the increase in steroids concentration leads to a higher synthesis of proteins and subsequent higher amount of muscular tissue, which needs, as a consequence, a higher volume of blood irrigating it and finally causing cardiovascular problems. High blood pressure could be observed also due to a regular administration of testosterone. In fact, such an administration causes a reduction in the secretion of HDL (High-Density Lipoproteins) resulting in an imbalance between HDL and LDL amounts leading to hypertension troubles. Other effects could be observed for female subjects submitted to a regular intake of AAS on hormonal cycle (ovulation and menstruation). The abuse affects also the psychological aspect and could lead to an aggressive attitude and even to depression.

4. Regulation

4.1 Bovine

The use of anabolic steroids as growth promoters in food-producing animals is prohibited in the European Union according to the EU Directive [5]. Different EU Directives have been issued to date in order to avoid any misuse of these substances in food-producing animals. The main purpose of these directives is to guarantee the security of the consumer toward these active chemicals [7].

The harmonization of the regulation concerning the use of these growth promoters in bovine, mainly between the European Union and the United States, has been problematic. The problem became even greater with the increase in the trade flows of bovine meat all over the world. While the use of anabolic steroids in the European Union is strictly banned in food-producing animals, the use of implants of 17β-testosterone, la 17β-estradiol, progesterone, trenbolone, or zeranol in cattle is still legal outside the European Union. As a consequence of the important position of the European Union in the bovine meat trade market, the bovine field in the United States witnessed a gradual decrease in the use of growth promoters. Although several arrangements have recently been taken in order to meet the different expectations of the different parties (MOU) (WT/DS26/28, September 30, 2009, 74 Federal Register), the problem is still persisting. In June 2013, talks between the European Union and the United States have been taken over in order to find a solution to this recurring issue. In July 2013, the TTIP "Transatlantic Trade and Investment Partnership," a project aiming to set a transatlantic market based on a liberal model ruled by a free circulation of goods and investments, was created. This project will also cover the agriculture field and would affect the regulation put into practice for the control of agricultural products such as bovine meat quality.

The recognized reference laboratories are submitted to the identification criteria established by the European Decisions 2002/657, which defines mainly the tolerated relative retention time and abundances percentual errors depending on the performed analytical technique.

4.2 Equine

The use of anabolic steroids is strictly banned in equestrian sports. Unlike WADA, where the list of prohibited substances for athletes is classified according to their respective pharmacological families, the IFHA has classified the doping substances for horses with regard to their respective target system of the organism. For instance, article 6 of IFHA "International Agreement on Breeding, Racing and Wagering" highlights the ban of substances that affect the nervous, the cardiovascular, the respiratory, the digestive, the urinary, the reproductive, the musculoskeletal, the blood, the immune, or the endocrine system.

The control of the use of these substances protects the integrity of horse races. This control can be conducted at any time of the year on a large panel of biological matrices.

With regard to the natural occurrence of some anabolic steroids such as nandrolone, the International Equestrian Federation put into practice in March 1988 an advisory committee formed of analysts and veterinarians, whose duty is to establish concentration or ratio thresholds of certain prohibited substances when it is necessary. Consequently, different confirmation thresholds have been approved by IFHA for natural occurring anabolic steroids misuse. For instance, boldenone urinary concentration should not overpass 15 ng/mL in entire male horses, testosterone urinary concentration should be inferior to 20 ng/mL in gelded horses and less than 55 ng/mL in mares and fillies. Finally, 5α-estrane-3β,17α-diol, one of the main recognized biomarkers of nandrolone administration, urinary concentration should be lower than 45 ng/mL in entire male horses [23]. In addition to the latter criterion, a complementary threshold consisting of a ratio of the urinary concentration of 5α-estrane-3β,17α-diol and 5(10)-estrene-3β,17α-diol of 1 has been supplemented [23].

The reference IFHA laboratories are submitted to the identification criteria established by AORC (Association of Official Racing Chemists), which defines mainly the tolerated retention time and relative abundances percentual errors depending on the analytical technique adopted [24].

5. The detection of steroid abuse in bovine and equine species

With regard to the high number of analysis performed by control laboratories, high-throughput screening analytical methods are required in order to offer a first discrimination between negative and suspicious samples. Once the sample is considered suspicious, it is subsequently submitted to confirmatory methods.

5.1 Screening

Screening methods require a dual compromising aspect by being high throughput and multi-residue but at the same time showing a high efficiency and low costs. These methods allow the detection or the concentration level estimation of a certain group of prohibited doping agents. Consequently, they affect a suspicious or a compliant status to the biological sample. These methods should present an as low as possible of "false positive" results and especially minimize the rate of "false negative" results (Decision 2002/657/EEC). These analytical techniques can either be immunological or based on chromatography coupled to mass spectrometry. The following synthesis review will highlight additionally novel analytical techniques, "omics" techniques, aiming at an indirect screening of prohibited substances, in particular natural occurring steroids.

5.1.1 Immunochemical techniques

Immunochemical techniques are based on an antigen-antibody interaction. There are two main techniques used: Radioimmunoassay (RIA), which is based on a radio element, and enzyme-linked immunosorbent assay (ELISA), which is based on an enzymatic system. These techniques permit the quantification of steroid hormones through the bindings established between their corresponding tracers, an analog of antigen, and the antibodies occurring in the biological sample. They classify hence the sample as compliant or suspicious. RIA needs a prior purification of the biological sample and offers several advantages, mainly the possibility to analyze different substances at once and to denature the sex hormone binding globulin (SHBG), which is transporting and bound to these substances. However, this tool requires large sample volumes especially when the substance is present at low concentration levels. It could also lead to erroneous results due to the reactivity of the antibody [25]. As for ELISA, it permits to measure the antigen through an enzymatic pathway. ELISA represented the reference tool for screening steroids abuse before the emergence of mass spectrometry tools. The main advantage of ELISA, in comparison with RIA, lies in the absence of a radio element tracer. However, ELISA exhibits lower specificity as compared with what can offer mass spectrometry.

5.1.2 Chromatography coupled to mass spectrometry

The analytical methods based on this technique allow identifying the administered substances or the markers resulting from such an administration. As far as endogenous AAS are concerned, this technique permits to give an idea about their concentration levels in the biological matrix in order to compare it with the settled thresholds. Two main branches of chromatography have been widely used for screening purposes: Gas Chromatography and Liquid Chromatography coupled to mass spectrometry.

5.1.2.1 Gas Chromatography-Mass Spectrometry (GC-MS)

GC-MS remains the most widespread technique used for screening analysis of steroid hormones in the anti-doping control laboratories [26, 27]. A sample preparation step consisting of a hydrolysis, extraction, concentration, and purification of the analytes is necessary in order to detect trace levels of substances of interest in the biological matrix. This technique usually requires a prior derivatization of the compounds with N-methyl-N-trimethylsilyl-trifluoroacetamide (MSTFA), PentaFluoroBenzaldehyde (PFB), or PentaFluoroPropionic Anhydride (PFPA) to enable their analysis on GC-MS. 5MS columns (5% phenyl and 95% of methylpolysiloxane) are usually used for chromatographic separation. Negative Chemical Ionization (NCI) and Electron Impact (EI) ionization modes are frequently used for analyses. Different analyzers have been used: ion trap [28], simple and triple quadripole [27, 29]. High-Resolution Mass spectrometry (HRMS) analyzers have also been used such as Time of Flight and Electromagnetic sector [29, 30].

The GC-MS techniques permit to obtain a better chromatographic separation than when operating with a Liquid Chromatography-Mass Spectrometry (LC-MS), even with the emergence of Ultra Performance Liquid Chromatography (UPLC). The main advantage of GC-MS, in comparison with LC-MS, is the absence of ion suppression effects.

GC-MS was in particular used for testosterone screening in equine species [31]. In bovine, GC-MS was used to figure out some potential biomarkers and thresholds for natural occurring steroids misuse. For instance, 5α-pregnane-3β,17α-diol was suggested as a biomarker for progesterone misuse, 5β-androstane-3α,17β-diol for testosterone misuse, 17β-androst-1-ene-3-one for boldenone misuse, and 17α-estradiol for estradiol misuse [32, 33].

New bidimensional separative techniques (GC × GC) have recently been reported in the anti-doping field [34]. The chromatographic separation on these systems is performed through two capillary columns placed in series permitting to obtain a higher separation power in comparison with unidimensional GC technique. In addition, the bidimensional gas chromatography results in a simplification of the sample preparation step by eliminating the purification process [35].

5.1.2.2 Liquid Chromatography-Mass Spectrometry (LC-MS)

LC-MS use in the anti-doping field as a screening technique has greatly increased with regard to the performance allowed [36]. LC-MS process results in a drastic gain of time in comparison with GC-MS technique regarding the lack of a derivatization step. Moreover, it enables the study of the conjugated form of the steroid in addition to its free form and therefore requires no hydrolysis step. This capacity allows a better understanding of the global metabolism of the steroids.

The ionization modes frequently used when dealing with AAS analyses in LC-MS are Atmospheric Pressure Chemical Ionization (APCI), Atmospheric Pressure Photo-Ionization (APPI), and Electrospray Ionization (ESI) [37]. The ionization type and mode depend strongly on the nature of the steroid. For instance, conjugated steroids are usually ionized in ESI^+ or ESI^- modes [38] and free steroid uniquely in ESI^+ mode.

In addition to the mass analyzers described previously for GC-MS analyses, LC offers the possibility to be coupled with other types of high-resolution mass analyzers such as Orbitrap or Fourier Transform Ion Cyclotron Resonance (FT-ICR) [39]. All of these analyzers offer the possibility to work with a high throughput, which is extremely important criterion for screening analyses [40, 41].

LC-MS was performed for screening purposes of more than 50 doping agents including testosterone, estradiol, boldenone, and norandrostenedione in porcine and bovine species [42]. It also detects fraudulent use of boldenone in bovine through the detection of the sulfoconjugated form [43]. In addition, it was performed in equine to detect testosterone, nandrolone, and boldenone misuse in entire male horses through the quantification of sulfoconjugated forms [44].

The emergence of UPLC permitted to improve the separation power of steroids and considerably reduced the analysis time. Different studies used this technique for AAS analysis and screening [45].

5.1.3 "Omic" techniques

"Omic" strategies have been applied in different scientific research fields mainly for biological applications. The "omic" techniques aim to study the recorded variations at different biological levels ranging from gene sequencing to metabolites expression [46]. It generates consequently a large amount of data permitting to understand the biological functioning of the organism as a whole. In the present context, the main objective of these approaches would be to determine biomarkers capable of characterizing the administration of a particular anabolic agent or a particular family of those agents [47]. These techniques have already shown their relevance in the anti-doping field, particularly, dealing with the issue of natural occurring steroids misuse. "Genomics" and "transcriptomics," "proteomics," and "metabolomics" have in particular been investigated to reveal candidate biomarkers that would serve screening purposes. Most of reported transcriptomic studies in the anti-doping field dealt with the influence of peptide hormones such as human Growth Hormone (hGH), Erythropoietin EPO and Insulin-like growth factor (IGF), and anabolic steroid hormones on the Deoxyribonucleic Acid (DNA) transcription [48–50]. These studies permitted to highlight some gene biomarkers.

The second strategy of interest in the cascade of "omics" (**Figure 3**) is "proteomics," which sheds the light on the proteome investigation. This approach is of high importance in the anti-doping field since permitting a profiling of the proteins concentration variations following the administration of anabolic substances [51]. Proteomics study may either be performed in an untargeted way or more targeted, focusing on a limited number of proteins of interest, a-priori selected. The untargeted proteomic study is usually performed in three main steps: first, the proteins are separated based on two-dimensional electrophoresis (2-DE) or multidimensional chromatography, then the analysis of the separated proteins is made by Matrix-Assisted Laser Desorption Ionization-Time Of Flight (MALDI-TOF) or MALDI-TOF/TOF, and finally, the proteins are identified. Very few untargeted proteomics works are reported in the field. However, several studies reported the use of targeted proteomics. For instance, Mooney confirmed the decrease of binding capacity of SHBG globulins in bovine following an administration of AAS [52]. In another study, Cacciatore demonstrated the variations occurring in concentration levels of IGF1, inhibins, and

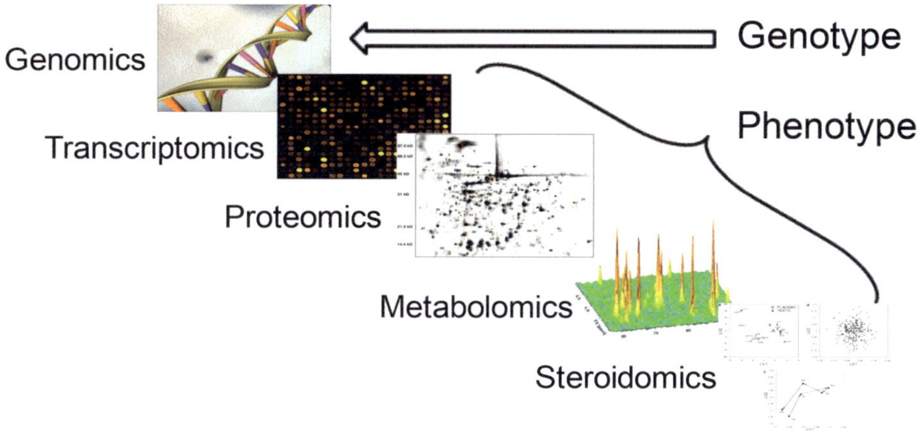

Figure 3.
" Omics " cascade.

osteocalcin after administration of estradiol and nandrolone [53]. In equine, Nagata confirmed a decrease in Luteinizing Hormone (LH) and inhibins concentration levels after an administration of nandrolone in stallions [54].

"Metabolomics" is the third family of interest in this "omics" family cascade. It focuses on the metabolome that is formed by the whole group of low-molecular-weight molecules. Sugar, organic acids, amino acids, vitamins, and steroids are part of the molecules included in metabolomic studies. Metabolomics consists of the study of the disturbance resulting from a genetic tampering of the organism or from a toxicological exposition or a treatment. The main objective of metabolomics is to shed light on compounds of interest potentially used to detect biological disturbance encountered by the organism. Many studies in the anti-doping field have evaluated this strategy, namely in human [55, 56], equine [57], or bovine [58, 59] species. These studies confirmed the feasibility and the efficiency of such an approach in this field. The different steps encountered for a metabolomic study are represented in **Figure 4**.

"Steroidomics," a subfamily of "Metabolomics," focuses on the study of the steroidome, the whole group of steroids in the organism. Steroidomics exhibits a similar analytical workflow as the one performed in metabolomics except that it focuses, through sample preparation and acquisition mode, on steroids monitoring [60]. It may be of interest in the anti-doping field, to study the variations of steroid concentration. This monitoring enables a better understanding of the consequences of anabolic steroids administration on AAS secretions in the organism. Consequently, a more accurate identification of doping cases with natural occurring steroids and an identification of potential candidate biomarkers are realized. This multidimensional approach mixing analytical and statistical tools requires an adequate sample preparation step and a specific detection method. Once the steroid profiles are obtained, they are submitted to a multivariate statistical processing to offer a first general view of the data distribution and the generated discrimination. Principal Components Analysis (PCA) and Orthogonal Partial Least Squares (OPLS) are two examples of, respectively, non-supervised and supervised statistical multivariate analysis tools. While PCA models permit to obtain a first overview of the sample distribution without any a priori instruction regarding their status, OPLS models are characterized by an incremented Y variable indicating the status of the sample and affecting a supervised nature to the model. Before proceeding to the statistical process of the

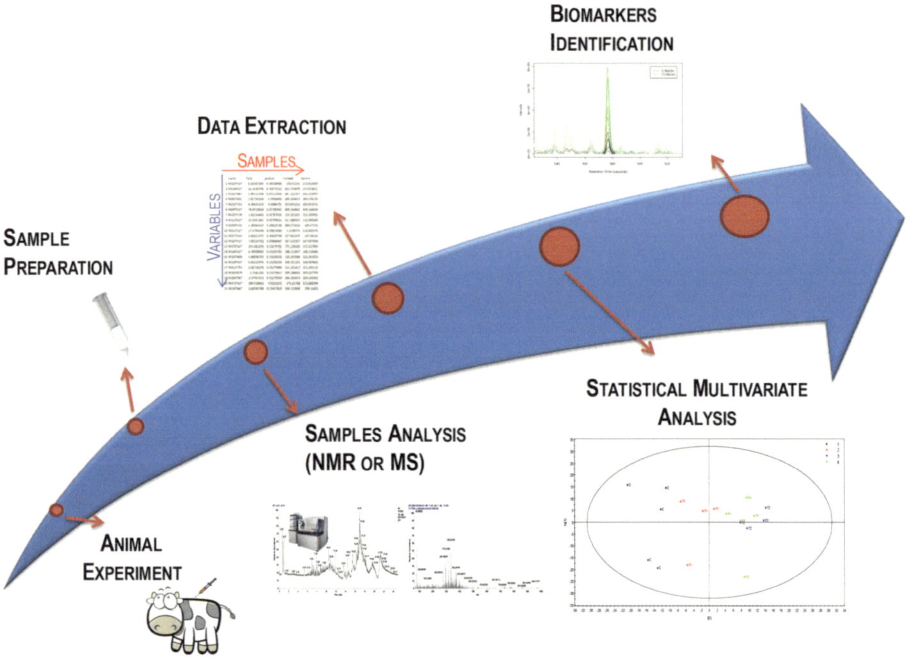

Figure 4.
The different steps of a metabolomic study.

data, the latter is normalized in order to decrease the statistical dominance of very intense peaks over less intense but interesting peaks. Finally, quality control samples, consisting of pools of the different samples of the study, should be injected all along the analyzed batches to assess the analytical robustness of the whole process and guarantee accurate analytical findings. Steroidomics can be divided in three main categories: non-targeted steroidomics, semi-targeted steroidomics, and targeted steroidomics. Non-targeted steroidomics requires a minimal sample preparation to avoid the loss of any steroid of interest. Rijk tested this technique to evidence many phase I and II steroid hormones biomarkers following testosterone precursors, DeHydroEpiAndrosterone (DHEA) and pregnenolone, administration in bovine [61]. Semi-targeted steroidomics consist of the assessment and monitoring of a specific fragment characterizing a group or a family of steroids. This approach has been used by Thevis, who discovered new synthetic steroids based on fragments at *m/z* 77, 91, and 105 corresponding respectively to fragments of steroids A ring and phenol group of estrogens [62]. In another study, Anizan selected fragment ions at m/z 97 and 113 to identify new sulfo and glucuruno-conjugated steroids attesting of an illegal administration of testosterone precursor, androstenedione, to bovine [63]. Finally, targeted steroidomics consists of the quantitative profiling of a selected set of steroids in order to study their concentration levels occurring variations following an anabolic treatment. Such a strategy was for example performed in order to establish suspicion thresholds and identify new biomarkers for DHEA, DiHydroTestosterone (DHT), and testosterone administration in men [64], to discriminate estradiol-treated bovine from the control group [65] and nandrolone-treated equine from control group [66] and served to evidence the evolution of steroid concentrations with regard to the seasonality [67].

5.2 Confirmatory strategies

The confirmation step is performed once the sample is declared suspicious following the screening process. The following part will review two main analytical approaches implemented to confirm natural AAS misuse.

5.2.1 Steroid esters detection

Steroid esters are synthetic compounds composed of a steroid moiety (the active part of the substance) and a side chain, which can be located on carbon 3 or more often on carbon 17 of the steroid. Since steroid esters are widely used in bovine and equine, several analytical strategies have already been developed to detect their misuse.

With regard to their lipophilic nature, the steroid esters cannot be detected in hydrophilic matrices such as urine. However, they can be detected in tissues [68], fat [69], hair [70], and blood [71].

While tissues and fat can only be collected at the slaughterhouse, hair and blood may be collected unambiguously from bovine and equine. Regarding hair, substances are actually transmitted to the hair through the hair follicle from blood stream or from sweat to the hair shaft. Hair can consequently provide a historical background on the steroid esters misuse. However, hair is a relatively complex matrix, and the analytical process adopted to extract substances from it is quite challenging. In fact, using harsh analytical conditions such as strong acidic or basic digestion of the hair can lead to the degradation of the ester. Instead, the use of soft analytical conditions such as methanolic extraction will result in a very low extraction recovery of the ester.

Taking into account these drawbacks, blood appears to be an interesting matrix with regard to its containment in steroid esters and the relatively easy analytical process to perform for extraction. The esters are transported through this matrix to the target cells and are usually bound to some blood proteins such as albumin [72] and SHBG [73]. These esters are gradually hydrolyzed in the blood stream by enzymatic esterase and are consequently found at trace levels (dozens to hundreds of pg/mL) [74]. Therefore, very sensitive analytical methods have been developed in order to detect them in blood [75] using some specific derivatization reactions in order to optimize the sensitivity [76, 77].

5.2.2 Isotopic approach

This approach consists of calculating isotopic ratios of different chemical elements such as $^{13}C/^{12}C$. This ratio can be expressed as an isotopic deviation following the application of the equation below:

$$\delta^{13}C[‰] = \left(\frac{\left(^{13}C/^{12}C\right)_{sample} - \left(^{13}C/^{12}C\right)_{standard}}{\left(^{13}C/^{12}C\right)_{standard}} \right) \times 10^3 \quad (1)$$

This ratio is measured based on a reference compound, the isotopic deviation of which is fixed at zero may be used for the purpose (e.g., Vienna Pee Dee Belemite (VPDB)).

In the anti-doping field, the purpose of this technique is to differentiate endogenous and exogenous anabolic steroids according to their enrichment in ^{13}C. The first applications involving the use of a GC-C-IRMS permitted to different anti-doping laboratories to identify exogenous testosterone in human [78–80]. This technique covered thereafter the animal anti-doping field and different studies using GC-C-IRMS focused on problematic issues related to the administration of natural steroids to equine [81] and bovine [82].

The small differences between endogenous and exogenous anabolic steroids isotopic deviations are one of the main difficulties encountered when applying the GC-Isotope Ratio Mass Spectrometry (IRMS) technique. In fact, the endogenous isotopic deviation of anabolic steroids depends mainly on the diet [83, 84]. Depending on the type of food consumed, the isotopic deviation of ingested cholesterol, and hence deriving anabolic steroids, will not be the same. Some plants called "C3 plants" such as wheat, rice, and soya exhibit low endogenous isotopic deviations in comparable ranges with those exhibited by synthetic steroids, mainly synthesized starting from C3 plants. However, the "C4 plants" such as maize and sugar cane generate a high endogenous isotopic deviation, which in this case of food-based diet permits to identify unambiguously exogenous administration of anabolic steroids.

6. Conclusion and perspectives

While the classical analytical methods, targeting a single or a large panel of anabolic substances, as currently implemented in the anti-doping and control laboratories are efficient to detect abuse with a large set of prohibited compounds, they have been showing some limits to detect abuse in some specific cases related to androgenic anabolic steroids misuse in racing and food producing animals. The difficulty has become even greater with the application of new doping methodologies aiming at bypassing the current analytical methods detection limits. The administrations of anabolic steroids cocktails, designer steroids, or natural occurring steroids are some examples of these new doping methodologies, which permit to escape control.

The use of natural occurring steroids such as testosterone appears to be one of the most challenging and problematic issues for doping control laboratories. With regard to their natural occurrence in the metabolism, the differentiation between their endogenous and exogenous origin becomes problematic. Moreover, the concentration levels of these steroid hormones vary between the different subjects part of the same species introducing inter-variability factors. Furthermore, these levels vary in the same subject at different time points due to different parameters such as seasonality, mating, and diet, which define the intra-variability factors. These two factors render the settling of a decision limit for a natural occurring steroid misuse difficult.

Testosterone in particular is among these steroids a problematic one for control laboratories since it has been shown to occur naturally in equine and bovine species while its administration under synthetic form is known to be very potent. Therefore, analytical strategies allowing to point out the exogenous administration are more than expected by the scientific community.

While confirmatory strategies seem to enable tackling the natural hormones issue and fulfill corresponding requirements, an additional effort appears necessary to validate the developed screening approach based on steroidomic profiling.

With regard to the general issue of natural steroids misuse in equine, more research work is needed in order to investigate minor metabolites of such administrations, which can reinforce the current international criteria. A stronger collaboration between the different reference laboratories worldwide is essential in order to settle population reference ranges of endogenous AAS and hence obtain a repository for future steroid doping challenges. A deeper investigation of the biosynthetic and physiological system of horses is also very important in order to have a better understanding of the biosynthetic pathway of endogenous steroids and hence generating a higher efficiency in tackling the issue.

Furthermore, other "upstream" omics techniques such as "genomic" and "transcriptomic" have been reported to be efficient for detecting natural steroids misuse and collaboration between these different fields would offer a mass global approach. For instance, Cannizzo developed a method based on DNA microarray data analysis [85] showing a large set of differentially expressed genes between controls and prednisolone treated bovine. Moreover, genomic instability and DNA damage were proven after nandrolone decanoate administration to rats [86]. However, such genotyping is costly in addition to the uneasiness of its application in the context of doping control. Many studies reported the possibility of generating information about the genotype starting from the phenotype and specifically steroid profiles [87–89]. These reported findings would offer a general overview of different organism levels and would be of a great help to evidence several challenging doping cases.

Author details

Zied Kaabia
GIE LCH, Verrières-le-Buisson, France

*Address all correspondence to: zied.kaabia@yahoo.fr

References

[1] Heitzman RJ. The effectiveness of anabolic agents in increasing rate of growth in farm animals; report on experiments in cattle. Environmental Quality and Safety. 1976;**5**:89-98

[2] Barceloux DG, Palmer RB. Anabolic—Androgenic steroids. Disease-a-Month. 2013;**59**:226-248

[3] Brown S. Note on the effects produced on man by subcutaneous injections of a liquid obtained from the testicles of animals. The Lancet. 1889;**134**:105-107

[4] Moran C, Quirke JF, Prendiville DJ, Bourke S, Roche JF. The effect of estradiol, trenbolone acetate, or zeranol on growth rate, mammary development, carcass traits, and plasma estradiol concentrations of beef heifers. Journal of Animal Science. 1991;**69**:4249-4258

[5] Council Directive 96/22/EC of 29 April 1996 concerning the prohibition on the use in stockfarming of certain substances having a hormonal or thyrostatic action and of ß-agonists, and repealing Directives 81/602/EEC, 88/146/EEC and 88/299/EEC

[6] Council Directive 96/23/EC of 29 April 1996 on measures to monitor certain substances and residues thereof in live animals and animal products and repealing Directives 89/187/EEC and 91/664/EEC

[7] Decision 2002/657/EEC CD, 2002. The Official Journal of European Communities

[8] Cantiello M, Carletti M, Cannizzo FT, Nebbia C, Bellino C, Pié S, et al. Effects of an illicit cocktail on serum immunoglobulins, lymphocyte proliferation and cytokine gene expression in the veal calf. Toxicology. 2007;**242**:39-51

[9] Scarth JP, Clarke AD, Teale P, Pearce CM. Comparative in vitro metabolism of the 'designer' steroid estra-4,9-diene-3,17-dione between the equine, canine and human: Identification of target metabolites for use in sports doping control. Steroids. 2010;**75**:643-652

[10] Catlin DH, Sekera MH, Ahrens BD, Starcevic B, Chang Y-C, Hatton CK. Tetrahydrogestrinone: Discovery, synthesis, and detection in urine. Rapid Communications in Mass Spectrometry. 2004;**18**:1245-1049

[11] Pitts SC, Davis M. An evidence-based analysis of anabolic steroids as performance enhancers in horses. Equine Veterinary Education. 2007;**19**:388-391

[12] Fajt VR, McCook C. An evidence-based analysis of anabolic steroids as therapeutic agents in horses. Equine Veterinary Education. 2008;**20**:542-544

[13] Fujioka M, Shinohara Y, Baba S, Irie M, Inoue K. Pharmacokinetic properties of testosterone propionate in norman men. Journal of Clinical Endocrinology & Metabolism. 1986;**63**:1361-1364

[14] Enever RP, Fotherby K, Naderi S, Lewis GA. Long-acting contraceptive agents: The influence of physicochemical properties of some esters of norethisterone upon the plasma levels of free norethisterone. Steroids. 1983;**41**:381-396

[15] Van der Vies J. Implications of basic pharmacology in the therapy with esters of nandrolone. Acta Edocrinologica Supplementum. 1985;**271**:38-44

[16] Stolker A, Groot M, Lasaroms J, Nijrolder A, Blokland M, Riedmaier I, et al. Detectability of testosterone esters and estradiol benzoate in bovine hair and plasma following pour-on treatment. Analytical and Bioanalytical Chemistry. 2009;**395**:1075-1087

[17] Tikkanen MJ, Vihma V, Jauhiainen M, Höckerstedt A, Helisten H, Kaamanen M. Lipoprotein-associated estrogens. Cardiovascular Research. 2002;**56**:184-188

[18] Hammond GL, Robinson PA, Sugino H, Ward DN, Finne J. Physicochemical characteristics of human sex hormone binding globulin: Evidence for two identical subunits. Journal of Steroid Biochemistry. 1986;**24**:815-824

[19] Lee IR, Greed LC, Hahnel R. Comparative measurements of plasma binding capacity and concentration of human sex hormone binding globulin. Clinica Chimica Acta. 1984;**137**:131-139

[20] Mangelsdorf DJ, Thummel C, Beato M, Herrlich P, Schütz G, Umesono K, et al. The nuclear receptor superfamily: The second decade. Cell. 1995;**83**:835-839

[21] Lehmann S. Etude de DAX-1 et de sa perte de fonction dans l'hypoplasie congénitale des glandes surrénales [PhD]. Strasbourg, France: Université Louis Pasteur Strasbourg I; 2005

[22] Van Amsterdam J, Opperhuizen A, Hartgens F. Adverse health effects of anabolic-androgenic steroids. Regulatory Toxicology and Pharmacology. 2010;**57**:117-123

[23] IFHA. International Agreement on Breeding, Racing and Wagering. Article 6. Paris, France: International Federation of Horseracing Authorities; 2022

[24] AORC. AORC Guidelines for the Minimum Criteria for Identification by Chromatography and Mass Spectrometry. Connecticut, USA: Association of Racing Chemists; 2016

[25] Stanczyk FZ, Clarke NJ. Advantages and challenges of mass spectrometry assays for steroid hormones. The Journal of Steroid Biochemistry and Molecular Biology. 2010;**121**:491-495

[26] Marcos J, Pascual JA, de la Torre X, Segura J. Fast screening of anabolic steroids and other banned doping substances in human urine by gas chromatography/tandem mass spectrometry. Journal of Mass Spectrometry. 2002;**37**:1059-1073

[27] De Brabander H, Van Gansbeke W, Geldof L, Van Eenoo P. An improved gas chromatography screening method for doping substances using triple quadrupole mass spectrometry, with an emphasis on quality assurance. Biomedical Chromatography. 2012;**26**:1416-1435

[28] Deventer K, Eenoo PV, Delbeke FT. Screening for anabolic steroids in doping analysis by liquid chromatography/electrospray ion trap mass spectrometry. Biomedical Chromatography. 2006;**20**:429-433

[29] Van Eenoo P, Van Gansbeke W, De Brabanter N, Deventer K, Delbeke FT. A fast, comprehensive screening method for doping agents in urine by gas chromatography–triple quadrupole mass spectrometry. Journal of Chromatography A. 2011;**1218**:3306-3316

[30] Revelsky AI, Samokhin AS, Virus ED, Rodchenkov GM, Revelsky IA. High sensitive analysis of steroids in doping control using gas chromatography/time-of-flight mass-spectrometry. Drug Testing and Analysis. 2011;**3**:263-267

[31] Yamada M, Aramaki S, Kurosawa M, Kijima-Suda I, Saito K, Nakazawa H. Simultaneous doping analysis of main urinary metabolites of anabolic steroids in horse by ion-trap gas chromatography-tandem mass spectrometry. Analytical Sciences. 2008;**24**:1199-1204

[32] Scarth JP, Clarke A, Teale P, Mill A, Macarthur R, Kay J. Detection of endogenous steroid abuse in cattle: Results from population studies in the UK. Food Additives & Contaminants: Part A. 2011;**28**:44-61

[33] Scarth JP, Kay J, Teale P, Akre C, Le Bizec B, De Brabander HF, et al. A review of analytical strategies for the detection of 'endogenous' steroid abuse in food production. Drug Testing and Analysis. 2012;**4**:40-49

[34] Mitrevski BS, Wilairat P, Marriott PJ. Comprehensive two-dimensional gas chromatography improves separation and identification of anabolic agents in doping control. Journal of Chromatography A. 2010;**1217**:127-135

[35] Zhang Y, Tobias HJ, Auchus RJ, Brenna JT. Comprehensive 2-dimensional gas chromatography fast quadrupole mass spectrometry (GC × GC-qMS) for urinary steroid profiling: Mass spectral characteristics with chemical ionization. Drug Testing and Analysis. 2011;**3**:857-867

[36] Noppe H, Le Bizec B, Verheyden K, De Brabander HF. Novel analytical methods for the determination of steroid hormones in edible matrices. Analytica Chimica Acta. 2008;**611**:1-16

[37] Jin Z, Daiya S, Kenttämaa HI. Characterization of nonpolar lipids and selected steroids by using laser-induced acoustic desorption/chemical ionization, atmospheric pressure chemical ionization, and electrospray ionization mass spectrometry. International Journal of Mass Spectrometry. 2011;**301**:234-239

[38] Kuuranne T, Vahermo M, Leinonen A, Kostiainen R. Electrospray and atmospheric pressure chemical ionization tandem mass spectrometric behavior of eight anabolic steroid glucuronides. Journal of the American Society for Mass Spectrometry. 2000;**11**:722-730

[39] Greig MJ, Bolaños B, Quenzer T, Bylund JMR. Fourier transform ion cyclotron resonance mass spectrometry using atmospheric pressure photoionization for high-resolution analyses of corticosteroids. Rapid Communications in Mass Spectrometry. 2003;**17**:2763-2768

[40] Liu Y, Uboh CE, Soma LR, Li X, Guan F, You Y, et al. Detection and confirmation of 60 anabolic and androgenic steroids in equine plasma by liquid chromatography-tandem mass spectrometry with instant library searching. Drug Testing and Analysis. 2011;**3**:54-67

[41] Wong CHF, Leung DKK, Tang FPW, Wong JKY, Yu NH, Wan TSM. Rapid screening of anabolic steroids in horse urine with ultra-high-performance liquid chromatography/tandem mass spectrometry after chemical derivatisation. Journal of Chromatography A. 2012;**1232**:257-265

[42] Yang Y, Shao B, Zhang J, Wu Y, Duan H. Determination of the residues of 50 anabolic hormones in muscle, milk and liver by very-high-pressure liquid chromatography-electrospray ionization tandem mass spectrometry. Journal of Chromatography B. 2009;**877**:489-496

[43] Destrez B, Bichon E, Rambaud L, Courant F, Monteau F, Pinel G, et al. Criteria to distinguish between natural

situations and illegal use of boldenone, boldenone esters and boldione in cattle: 2. Direct measurement of 17β-boldenone sulpho-conjugate in calf urine by liquid chromatography–high resolution and tandem mass spectrometry. Steroids. 2008;**74**:803-808

[44] Grace PB, Drake EC, Teale P, Houghton E. Quantification of 19-nortestosterone sulphate and boldenone sulphate in urine from male horses using liquid chromatography/tandem mass spectrometry. Rapid Communications in Mass Spectrometry. 2008;**22**:2999-3007

[45] Mazzarino M, Botrè F. A fast liquid chromatographic/mass spectrometric screening method for the simultaneous detection of synthetic glucocorticoids, some stimulants, anti-oestrogen drugs and synthetic anabolic steroids. Rapid Communications in Mass Spectrometry. 2006;**20**:3465-3476

[46] Nicholson JK, Holmes E, Elliott P. The metabolome-wide association study: A new look at human disease risk factors. Journal of Proteome Research. 2008;**7**:3637-3638

[47] Riedmaier I, Becker C, Pfaffl MW, Meyer HHD. The use of omic technologies for biomarker development to trace functions of anabolic agents. Journal of Chromatography A. 2009;**1216**:8192-8199

[48] Bailly-Chouriberry L, Pinel G, Garcia P, Popot M-A, Le Bizec B, Bonnaire Y. Identification of recombinant equine growth hormone in horse plasma by LC–MS/MS: A confirmatory analysis in doping control. Analytical Chemistry. 2008;**80**:8340-8347

[49] Riedmaier I, Tichopad A, Reiter M, Pfaffl MW, Meyer HHD. Identification of potential gene expression biomarkers for the surveillance of anabolic agents in bovine blood cells. Analytica Chimica Acta. 2009;**638**:106-113

[50] Riedmaier I, Pfaffl MW. Transcriptional biomarkers—High throughput screening, quantitative verification, and bioinformatical validation methods. Methods. 2013;**59**:3-9

[51] Cunningham MJ. Genomics and proteomics: The new millennium of drug discovery and development. Journal of Pharmacological end Toxicological Methods. 2000;**44**:291-300

[52] Mooney MH, Bergwerff AA, van Meeuwen JA, Luppa PB, Elliott CT. Biosensor-based detection of reduced sex hormone-binding globulin binding capacities in response to growth-promoter administrations. Analytica Chimica Acta. 2009;**637**:235-240

[53] Cacciatore G, Eisenberg SWF, Situ C, Mooney MH, Delahaut P, Klarenbeek S, et al. Effect of growth-promoting 17β-estradiol, 19-nortestosterone and dexamethasone on circulating levels of nine potential biomarker candidates in veal calves. Analytica Chimica Acta. 2009;**637**:351-359

[54] Nagata S, Kurosawa M, Mima K, Nambo Y, Fujii Y, Watanabe G, et al. Effects of anabolic steroid (19-nortestosterone) on the secretion of testicular hormones in the stallion. Journal of Reproduction and Fertility. 1999;**115**:373-379

[55] Fiehn O. Metabolomics—The link between genotypes and phenotypes. Plant Molecular Biology. 2002;**48**:155-171

[56] Fiehn O. Extending the breadth of metabolite profiling by gas chromatography coupled to mass spectrometry. TrAC Trends in Analytical Chemistry. 2008;**27**:261-269

[57] Cloteau C, Dervilly G, Kaabia Z, Bagilet F, Delcourt V, Loup B, et al. From a non-targeted metabolomics approach to a targeted biomarkers strategy to highlight testosterone abuse in equine. Illustration of a methodological transfer between platforms and laboratories. Drug Testing and Analysis. 2022;**14**(5):864-878

[58] Courant F, Pinel G, Bichon E, Monteau F, Antignac J-P, Le Bizec B. Development of a metabolomic approach based on liquid chromatography-high resolution mass spectrometry to screen for clenbuterol abuse in calves. Analyst. 2009;**134**:1637-1646

[59] Anizan S, Bichon E, Duval T, Monteau F, Cesbron N, Antignac J-P, et al. Gas chromatography coupled to mass spectrometry-based metabolomic to screen for anabolic practices in cattle: Identification of 5α-androst-2-en-17-one as new biomarker of 4-androstenedione misuse. Journal of Mass Spectrometry. 2012;**47**:131-140

[60] Kaabia Z, Laparre J, Dervilly-Pinel G, Mooney M, Buckley T, Sherry M, et al. Comprehensive steroid profiling by liquid chromatography coupled to high resolution mass spectrometry. The Journal of Steroid Biochemistry and Molecular Biology. 2018;**183**:106-115

[61] Rijk JCW, Lommen A, Essers ML, Groot MJ, Van Hende JM, Doeswijk TG, et al. Metabolomics approach to anabolic steroid urine profiling of bovines treated with prohormones. Analytical Chemistry. 2009;**81**:6879-6888

[62] Thevis M, Bommerich U, Opfermann G, Schänzer W. Characterization of chemically modified steroids for doping control purposes by electrospray ionization tandem mass spectrometry. Journal of Mass Spectrometry. 2005;**40**:494-502

[63] Anizan S, Di Nardo D, Bichon E, Monteau F, Cesbron N, Antignac J-P, et al. Targeted phase II metabolites profiling as new screening strategy to investigate natural steroid abuse in animal breeding. Analytica Chimica Acta. 2011;**700**:105-113

[64] Van Renterghem P, Van Eenoo P, Sottas P-E, Saugy M, Delbeke F. Subject-based steroid profiling and the determination of novel biomarkers for DHT and DHEA misuse in sports. Drug Testing and Analysis. 2010;**2**:582-588

[65] Regal P, Nebot C, Díaz-Bao M, Barreiro R, Cepeda A, Fente C. Disturbance in sex-steroid serum profiles of cattle in response to exogenous estradiol: A screening approach to detect forbidden treatments. Steroids. 2011;**76**:365-375

[66] Kaabia Z, Dervilly-Pinel G, Popot MA, Bailly-Chouriberry L, Plou P, Bonnaire Y, et al. Monitoring the endogenous steroid profile disruption in urine and blood upon nandrolone administration: An efficient and innovative strategy to screen for nandrolone abuse in entire male horses. Drug Testing and Analysis. 2014;**6**:376-388

[67] Moeller B, Brown S, Pierce S, Van Balen C, Stanley S. Endogenous steroid profiling of young thoroughbred horses in athletic training. In: Proceedings of the 55th Annual Convention of the American Association of Equine Practitioners; December 5-9, 2009; Las Vegas, Nevada. Vol. 55. Nevada, USA: American Association of Equine Practitioners; 2009. p. 317

[68] Hochberg RB. Biological esterification of steroids. Endocrinology Reviews. 1998;**19**:331-348

[69] Badeau M, Vihma V, Mikkola TS, Tiitinen A, Tikkanen MJ. Estradiol fatty acid esters in adipose tissue

and serum of pregnant and pre- and postmenopausal women. The Journal of Clinical Endocrinology and Metabolism. 2007;**92**:4327-4331

[70] Nielen MWF, Lasaroms JJP, Mulder PPJ, Van Hende J, van Rhijn JA, Groot MJ. Multi residue screening of intact testosterone esters and boldenone undecylenate in bovine hair using liquid chromatography electrospray tandem mass spectrometry. Journal of Chromatography B. 2006;**830**:126-134

[71] Kaabia Z, Dervilly-Pinel G, Hanganu F, Cesbron N, Bichon E, Popot MA, et al. Ultra high performance liquid chromatography/tandem mass spectrometry based identification of steroid esters in serum and plasma: An efficient strategy to detect natural steroids abuse in breeding and racing animals. Journal of Chromatography A. 2013;**1284**:126-140

[72] Burton R, Westphal U. Steroid hormone-binding proteins in blood plasma. Metabolism. 1972;**21**:253-276

[73] Dunn J, Nisula B, Rodbard D. Transport of steroid hormones: Binding of 21 endogenous steroids to both testosterone-binding globulin and corticosteroid-binding globulin in human plasma. The Journal of Clinical Endocrinology and Metabolism. 1981;**53**:58-68

[74] Bischoff F, Yee YS, Moran JJ, Katherman RE. Enzymatic hydrolysis of steroid hormone esters by blood serum. The Journal of Biological Chemistry. 1951;**189**:729-738

[75] Shackleton CHL, Chuang H, Kim J, de la Torre X, Segura J. Electrospray mass spectrometry of testosterone esters: Potential for use in doping control. Steroids. 1997;**62**:523-529

[76] Kirk JM, Tarbin J, Keely BJ. Analysis of androgenic steroid Girard P hydrazones using multistage tandem mass spectrometry. Rapid Communications in Mass Spectrometry. 2006;**20**:1247-1252

[77] Gray BP, Teale P, Pearce CM. Analysis of methyloxime derivatives of intact esters of testosterone and boldenone in equine plasma using ultra high performance liquid chromatography tandem mass spectrometry. Drug Testing and Analysis. 2011;**3**:206-213

[78] Southan G, Mallat A, Jumeau J, Craig S, Poojara N, Mitchell D. Programme and Abstracts of the Second International Symposium on Applied Mass Spectrometry in the Health Sciences. Barcelona: Biomedical & Environmental Mass Spectrometry; 1990. p. 360

[79] Becchi M, Aguilera R, Farizon Y, Flament MM, Casabianca H, James P. Gas chromatography/combustion/isotope-ratio mass spectrometry analysis of urinary steroids to detect misuse of testosterone in sport. Rapid Communication in Mass Spectrometry. 1994;**8**:304-308

[80] Aguilera R, Becchi M, Casabianca H, Hatton CK, Catlin DH, Starcevic B, et al. Improved method of detection of testosterone abuse by gas hromatography/combustion/isotope ratio mass spectrometry analysis of urinary steroids. Journal of Mass Spectrometry. 1996;**31**:169-176

[81] Aguilera R, Becchi M, Mateus L, Popot MA, Bonnaire Y, Casabianca H, et al. Detection of exogenous hydrocortisone in horse urine by gas chromatography–combustion–carbon isotope ratio mass spectrometry. Journal of Chromatography B: Biomedical Sciences and Applications. 1997;**702**:85-91

[82] Ferchaud V, Le Bizec B, Monteau F, Andre F. Determination of the exogenous character of testosterone in bovine urine by gas chromatography-combustion-isotope ratio mass spectrometry[dagger]. Analyst. 1998;**123**:2617-2620

[83] Ferchaud V, Le Bizec B, Monteau F, Andre F. Characterization of exogenous testosterone in livestock by gas chromatography/combustion/isotope ratio mass spectrometry: Influence of feeding and age. Rapid Communications in Mass Spectrometry. 2000;**14**:652-656

[84] Saudan C, Kamber M, Barbati G, Robinson N, Desmarchelier A, Mangin P, et al. Longitudinal profiling of urinary steroids by gas chromatography/combustion/isotope ratio mass spectrometry: Diet change may result in carbon isotopic variations. Journal of Chromatography B. 2006;**831**:324-327

[85] Cannizzo FT, Pegolo S, Starvaggi Cucuzza L, Bargelloni L, Divari S, Franch R, et al. Gene expression profiling of thymus in beef cattle treated with prednisolone. Research in Veterinary Science. 2013;**95**:540-547

[86] Pozzi R, Fernandes K, Moura C, Ferrari R, Fernandes K, Renno A, et al. Nandrolone decanoate induces genetic damage in multiple organs of rats. Archives of Environmental Contamination and Toxicology. 2013;**64**:514-518

[87] Malin B, Sweeney L. Inferring genotype from clinical phenotype through a knowledge based algorithm. Pacific Symposium on Biocomputing. 2002:41-52

[88] Prank K, Schulze E, Eckert O, Nattkemper TW, Bettendorf M, Maser-Gluth C, et al. Machine learning approaches for phenotype–genotype mapping: Predicting heterozygous mutations in the CYP21B gene from steroid profiles. European Journal of Endocrinology. 2005;**153**:301-305

[89] Schulze J, Rane A, Ekstrom L. Genetic variation in androgen disposition: Implications in clinical medicine including testosterone abuse. Expert Opinion on Drug Metabolism & Toxicology. 2009;**5**:731-744

Chapter 4

Evolutionary Theory of an Association between Testosterone and Attractiveness Perception in Humans

Hirokazu Doi

Abstract

Literature on psychological function of testosterone in humans has emphasized its association with such traits as aggressiveness and impulsivity. In addition, increasing number of studies have shown the linkage between testosterone level and individual difference in the strength of preference for other's sexually dimorphic traits. According to theorists in the field of evolutionary psychology, the preference pattern for sexual dimorphisms had evolved as an adaptive mechanism to increase the odds of reproductive success. But, so far, there are few systematic syntheses of literatures to validate such evolutionary explanation from the perspective of androgenic function. This chapter aims to give an overview of the existing findings on the association between testosterone and preference pattern in humans and discuss their implications for evolutionary explanation of human attractiveness perception.

Keywords: testosterone, preference, face, voice, evolutionary psychology

1. Introduction

Numerous functions of the central nervous system, perception, motor control, emotion, homeostatic balance, and so on, are discussed in the literature on psychology. The neurophysiological machinery for many of these psychological and cognitive functions has probably evolved as an adaptive mechanism—or at least as a by-product of adaptive mechanisms—to meet the demands of survival in a given environment.

The endocrinological function is tightly intertwined with neural—and hence, psychological—and cognitive functions. For example, in the cascade of fear response, the amygdala initiates a cascade process in the hypothalamic–pituitary–adrenal (HPA) axis, leading to the secretion of glucocorticoids in the adrenal gland, thereby enhancing energy consumption [1, 2]. An important implication of this is that individual differences within the endocrinological function are possibly linked to diversity in psychological traits and responses.

In addition to its physiological actions, testosterone has long been associated with psychological traits such as aggressiveness [3, 4] and impulsivity [5], especially in males. Empirical studies using a pen-and-pencil questionnaire or well-tested paradigms of behavioral measurement have shown that people with high circulating testosterone levels tend to show more aggressive [3, 4] and dominant behavior [6]. Several earlier studies have identified a positive relationship between testosterone levels and trait impulsivity. At the same time, even when using a similar behavioral paradigm, studies have often reported mixed results as for the association between impulsivity and testosterone level, which indicates intrinsic complexity in androgenic influences on human behavior. For example, our study [7] found sex differences in the association between salivary testosterone levels and impulsivity in financial decision making, which indicates non-linearity in the pattern of influence of testosterone on a few domains of cognitive function (see also [8, 9]).

Attractiveness is among the primary attributes that determine first impressions, and attractive people make good impressions in job interviews [10, 11], receive priority in promotion [12]—possibly through a halo effect ([13, 14] but see [15])—and, importantly, in the context of this chapter, are more likely to have many sexual partners [16, 17].

In contrast to the common sense that beauty and attractiveness are defined by cultural standards, studies in the past three decades have shown the possibility that some physical traits are universally perceived to be attractive and that hormones, including testosterone, play pivotal roles in shaping attractive features and determining the strength of one's preference for them. This chapter aims to give a brief overview of the previous findings on the link between testosterone and human attractiveness perception and discuss the validity of evolutionary explanations for the observed associations.

2. Androgenic regulation of reproductive behavior

Reproduction is, in a sense, the ultimate goal of living organisms—both as individuals and as members of one's own species. In addition to other hormones, testosterone and its metabolites are integrated into the complex web of the neuroendocrine system that controls the reproductive process.

Testosterone plays a pivotal role in the regulation of the male reproductive system; it controls male masculinization in body morphology and physiology [18–20] and sexual behavior [21] in variety of species. The concentration of androgen is much higher in the testes than in the bloodstream, and spermatogenesis is highly dependent on this high level of testicular testosterone [22].

There are a few controversies regarding the role of testosterone in the female reproductive process. However, at least in vitro, several studies have shown that testosterone and its metabolites promote the early stages of ovarian follicular maturation [23] directly as well as via conversion to estrogen through aromatization.

In addition to these physiological effects, several studies have shown that testosterone can modulate the function of the central nervous system, resulting in multiple aspects of reproductive behavior. Circulating testosterone levels are positively associated with male aggression, intra-sex competitiveness, and sexual desire in non-human species [21], which increases the success rate of winning and sexual intercourse with female conspecifics. In accordance with these observations, human studies have also supported the relationship between sexual desire and testosterone levels in both males [24] and females [25].

Maintaining a higher social status leads to an increased likelihood of reproductive success. Testosterone levels have been suggested to modulate the higher-order cognitive process of status seeking behavior. Eisenberger reported that men administered with testosterone make fairer offers in economic bargaining than placebo [26] and are more likely to punish those who make unfair offers [27]; both behaviors are beneficial for elevating one's social status. Likewise, exogenous testosterone administration increases generosity when the audience is observing one's behavior [28], which probably contributes to keeping good reputation.

Recent studies have shown that, in addition to its association with sexual behavior, testosterone levels modulate paternal investment. A longitudinal study [29] showed a reduction in testosterone levels in males after the delivery of their first child, similar to the findings in marmosets. Moreover, the time spent on care-taking was negatively correlated with testosterone levels. In a laboratory study [30], new fathers with low serum testosterone levels showed empathic responses more strongly to the sounds of the infant's cry. These studies indicate a suppressive effect of circulating testosterone on paternal investment.

3. Evolutionary theory of attractiveness

Mainly two types of explanations can be distinguished [31, 32] for certain behaviors or behavioral tendencies observed in animals: proximate and ultimate. The first refers to the description of biological mechanisms underlying animal behavior, such as neural functions and physiological responses. In the case of attractiveness perception, viewing attractive others activates the neural network of the reward system and induces pleasure [33]. This hedonic state is considered to promote the favorable treatment of physically attractive people.

The ultimate explanation of a behavior answers such questions as what kind of adaptive benefit and costs the behavior of interest incurs and how the behavior has evolved. The possession of eye-catching ornaments in certain species, such as the long tail in peacocks, has been a puzzle for evolutionary theorists. Conspicuous tails of peacocks are almost useless in themselves and could jeopardize the survival of a peacock by making it easily detectable by predators. Why did this phenotype evolve in the first place? This question explains the evolutionary roots of sexually dimorphic traits in peacocks.

The costly signaling theory (or good-genes handicap principle) claims that possession of extravagant ornaments functions as an "honest signal" of an individual's health and reproductive prowess [34, 35]. Production and sustainment of the long tail in peacocks is energy consuming and, as mentioned above, has the potential to lower the odds of survival. This indicates that a male with a long tail is healthy and strong enough to survive despite such a large handicap. In this line of reasoning, it follows that it is an adaptive strategy for peahens in bearing offsprings with "good genes" by mating with peacocks with long tails, because a long tail is an honest signal of biological quality. Though controversial, some ethological and experimental studies obtained several pieces of supporting evidence that males with seemingly maladaptive morphological traits achieve higher reproductive success [36–38].

The role of testosterone in the perception of attractiveness is often explained based on its value of signaling. Given the association between androgen and the male reproductive function [18–22, 37, 38], morphological traits linked to high levels of testosterone can serve as a signal of high reproductivity.

Another type of testosterone signaling function has also been suggested, based on the observation that testosterone suppresses the immune response to stressors. Based on this observation, a high level of testosterone can be deemed a handicap in the survival of an organism. Thus, the immunocompetence handicap theory [39, 40] of testosterone claims that morphological traits indicative of high testosterone levels advertise high immunocompetence and higher function of the immunological system because only individuals with strong immunity can survive despite the immunosuppressive effect of testosterone.

These hypotheses claim that masculine morphological traits function as an honest signal of biological quality and fitness of an individual and thus indicate the signaling quality of these traits as an ultimate explanation of why females are attracted to masculine traits in males. Females who are attracted to masculine males mate with a high-quality male, which probably increases the odds of offspring survival. Through sexual selection, traits indicative of high androgen levels have been consolidated in male sexual dimorphism, and the female neural system has evolved to be predisposed to seek males with these traits as mating partners.

4. Association between testosterone and attractiveness perception

To evaluate the validity of these evolutionary theories of attractive phenotypes, a good starting point is the examination of existing findings on human attractiveness perception. Over the past three decades, scores of studies have been published on the characteristics of sensory signals that young adult males and females find attractive; many of these studies have dealt with the attractiveness perception of sexual dimorphism in face and voice. These studies generally indicate that certain facial and vocal traits are universally perceived as attractive. Additionally, in line with the proverb "beauty lies in the eyes of the beholder," there is notable intra- and inter-individual differences in the strength of preference depending on the hormonal state. According to several researchers, the pattern of attractiveness perception and findings on the endocrinological basis of individual differences in attractiveness perception provide at least partial support for evolutionary theory of attractiveness perception.

4.1 Faces

The face is among the most prominent sources of social information, and the human visual system is equipped to extract various kinds of information from others' faces. When female faces are presented side by side, infants as young as two months old spend more time looking at female faces that are evaluated to be more beautiful by adults [41]. Although the ability to capture attention is an inherently different concept from attractiveness, this finding indicates that facial attractiveness may comprise a collection of low-level perceptual features that can be processed by an immature brain.

Studies of young adults have identified facial asymmetry as a strong determinant of perceived facial attractiveness. Fluctuating asymmetry is a random deviation from perfect symmetry in the body and is presumed to reflect an organism's susceptibility to stressors; thus, the lower the fluctuating asymmetry an individual exhibits, the more physically fit he/she is. Previous studies have generally agreed that a low level of fluctuating asymmetry is perceived to be attractive regardless of the face model and evaluator's sex [42, 43] (but see [44]).

Another type of morphological feature that is universally perceived as attractive is the so-called baby schema ("Kindchenschema" [45]). Infants of many species share a collection of similar morphological traits such as large eyes, round contours, and small noses. Baby schema is asserted to function as a releaser of caretaking behaviors of adult conspecifics [46]. Glocker et al. [47] showed that a computer-synthesized infant face with its "baby schema" exaggerated activates the reward region more vigorously than the original image. Attractiveness perception in baby schema is seemingly influenced by the endocrinological function. Hahn et al. [48] revealed that intra-individual fluctuation in rewarding value one finds in a baby's face is dependent on testosterone levels. Testosterone works in concert with oxytocin to modulate the responses of infants' faces. A behavioral study [49] revealed that nulliparous women with high testosterone levels are slower in detecting infant faces than those with low testosterone levels. However, the reaction time to infant face was accelerated by exogenous administration of oxytocin, most prominently in women with high testosterone levels.

Certain adults strongly exhibit baby schemas on their faces. Studies in the field of social psychology have revealed that people implicitly project infant-like traits such as innocence and incompetence [50, 51]. In our study [52], which investigated neural substrates linked to this over-generalization of baby schema to adult faces, part of the ventral striatum was more strongly activated to babyish than the mature version of an identical face. Part of the inter-individual variance in this activation was explained by the oxytocin level; however, in contrast to the case of infant face, testosterone was not identified as a determinant of reward system activation to faces of baby-faced adults.

In contrast to the case of low fluctuating asymmetry and baby schema that are almost universally perceived to be attractive [42, 43, 46, 52], the attractiveness perception of sexual dimorphisms in the human face is dependent on both the model's and the rater's sex. Sexual dimorphism refers to morphological features exaggerated in one sex. In the case of the human face, sexual dimorphisms in prototypical male faces include masculine features, such as large jawbones, protruded eyebrows, angular facial contours, and thinner lips, whereas feminine features are characterized by morphological features exaggerated in the opposite direction.

As can be intuitively understood, females with more feminine faces are perceived as more attractive than masculine ones [53] (but see [54]). If feminine features in female faces are exploited as signals of fecundity, it follows that preference for feminine faces is particularly prominent in male viewers compared to female viewers. This conjecture is supported in many studies [53, 55, 56], but some argue that there is considerable variation among males in the strength of preference for feminine female faces depending on self-perceived attractiveness and mating strategy [57, 58].

Another line of study found a positive association between circulating testosterone levels and the degree of male preference for femininity in female faces [59]. The results of correlational studies are further bolstered by the finding of a causal relationship between testosterone levels and perceived attractiveness in feminine morphological features. Welling et al. showed that winning in competition enhances male preference for female faces' femininity [60]. Although they did not directly measure testosterone concentration, this finding hints at the possibility that testosterone level is causally linked to the attractiveness perception of female sexual dimorphism in males because winning in competition is known to result in phasic testosterone increase [61]. More direct evidence for causal linkage comes from testosterone administration studies that the administration of a testosterone patch increases preference for feminine faces [62]. At the same time, another administration study reported a contradictory result that exogenous administration of testosterone decreases preference for femininity in female faces in a long-term relationship context [63].

The observed pattern of attractiveness perception of masculine facial features was somewhat complicated. In contrast to feminine female faces, which are judged to be attractive by both males and females alike [53], masculine male faces are not unequivocally perceived to be more attractive than less-masculine faces [64, 65]. One plausible reason for this observation is that masculine features are coupled with the impressions of dominance and untrustworthiness [53].

Sex hormones engender variations in females' perceptions of attractiveness in masculine male faces at both inter- and intra-individual levels. One correlational study has reported that females with high estradiol level show stronger preference for male faces with high testosterone [66]. A seminal study by Penton-Voak et al. [67] revealed cyclic fluctuations in the preference for masculine and feminine versions of a male face across the menstrual cycle. More specifically, during late follicular and ovulatory phase with high conception risk, females preferred masculine over feminine versions of identical male faces for partner of short-term relationship more than during the luteal phase with low conception risk. Several later studies successfully replicated this "ovulatory shift" pattern in females' perceptions of attractiveness in masculine facial features [66, 68, 69]. One interpretation of the ovulatory shift is that fluctuations in facial preference across the menstrual cycle are dependent on the mating strategy [66]. During the late follicular to ovulatory phase, females seek to find sexual partner with "good genes" to bear offspring with the greatest chance of survival, which makes them prefer masculine features. Testosterone levels are often linked to poor parental investment in fathers [29, 30]. Thus, it is a good strategy for females to mate with males with feminine morphology, from whom they can expect greater effort in parenting during the luteal phase. Partial support for the association between mating strategy and masculinity preference in females is obtained in several studies. For example, Roney et al. [70] reported that females rated male faces with high interest in children and those with high masculinity more attractive as long- and short-term partners, respectively (see also [71]). Menstrual cycle is accompanied by cyclic change in levels of multiple hormones. Consistently, several studies found a relationship between facial masculinity preference and estradiol [66] and progesterone [69] (but see [72, 73]). Testosterone level also fluctuates during menstrual cycle [74, 75]. This observation raises the possibility that facial masculinity preferences is also linked to testosterone level in females, but previous studies reported mixed findings as for this conjecture [71, 76, 77].

It should be noted that the phenomenon of cyclic shift in facial masculinity preference and its "mating strategy" interpretation are far from established in its current state. Many methodological problems have been pointed out in the studies on cyclic shift in face preference [78]. Several empirical studies reported no difference in masculinity preference between high and low conception risk phases during menstrual cycle [73] or lack of association between hormonal status and masculinity preference [72] (see [78] for a brief review). One study even reported that females preferred faces of males with relatively low level of serum testosterone during the fertile phase of menstrual cycle [79] in direct contradiction to the widespread interpretation.

4.2 Voices

Prominent sexual dimorphisms in human voices become clearly observable after puberty, during which the morphology of the vocal tract undergoes maturational changes [80] under hormonal influences [81]. Sexual dimorphism in voice expresses itself through two main aspects: fundamental frequency and formant dispersion [82, 83]. The fundamental frequency of a voice is the frequency at which the vocal fold vibrates, and its perceptual correlation is the pitch. Formant refers to the local zenith in the frequency in power distribution, where the power within specific frequency ranges is amplified by resonance in the vocal tract. The combination of formant frequencies determines the perceived vowel category.

Fundamental frequency is lower in males than in females [82]. Similarly, formant dispersion, which is the frequency distance between neighboring formants, is narrower in males [84], and spacing between formants is related to body size in macaques [85] though the relationship is relatively weak in humans [86]. Based on these observations, many experimental studies have focused on the association between these vocal features and voice impressions. As in the case of facial masculinity, voices with muscular features, low fundamental frequency, and narrow formant dispersion give an impression of dominance [87]. A male's voice with a low fundamental and formant frequency is evaluated as more attractive by females than that with a high frequency [88, 89]. Likewise, males prefer female voices with high fundamental frequency and wide formant dispersion [90]. One explanation for such pattern of preference is that acoustic characteristics of voice reflect body size and physical function of speakers; females prefer males with voice indicative of a large body size [91, 92] and physical strength [93]. A recent study [83] has identified a curvilinear relationship between perceived attractiveness and fundamental/formant frequency: overall, male voices with low fundamental frequency tended to be rated higher in attractiveness. Interestingly, this effect was particularly pronounced when female raters evaluated voice attractiveness in a short-term rather than in a long-term context, closely replicating the pattern observed in face attractiveness studies [94]. Outside of the laboratory, it has been shown that males—but not females—with a low-pitched voice succeed in bearing a greater number of children [95].

Relatively less research has been conducted on whether hormonal status modulates the attractiveness perception of sexually dimorphic traits in voices, and we are yet to obtain a coherent picture regarding this issue. A few studies found cyclic variation in masculine traits in male's voice across menstrual cycle [84, 96], especially in females with low trait estradiol level [84]. Pisanski et al. [97] have linked intra-individual fluctuation in females' preference for masculine traits in men's voice to female's salivary level of estradiol rather than progesterone or testosterone. In males, Kandrik et al. [98] failed to find any association between attractiveness perception in feminine voices and testosterone levels.

5. Signal value of sexual dimorphisms

Although still equivocal, previous research has found some pieces of evidence supporting evolutionary theory of attractiveness perception. Another important aspect to be considered in validating the signaling hypothesis is whether attractive traits actually signal qualities advantageous for reproduction and offspring survival. Although this number is disproportionally small compared to purely psychological and observational studies that address the pattern and mechanism of attractiveness perception, researchers have made progress in empirically validating the signal value of attractive features.

The activational effect of androgens has been shown to contribute to cranial growth [99] and vocal apparatus maturation [80]. Consistently, previous studies have revealed an association between the expression of masculine traits and testosterone levels in facial morphology [100] and acoustic features of voice [83, 101]. However, linking muscular features and reproductive processes in males is not straightforward. Few studies have empirically investigated the relationship between reproductive function and masculine traits. A pioneering study by Soler et al. [102] reported a positive association between facial attractiveness and semen quality, as assessed by sperm motility and morphology. However, later studies failed to replicate the predicted association between semen quality, attractiveness, and masculinity in the face [103] and voice [104].

The immunocompetence handicap theory of testosterone asserts that men with high testosterone levels possess strong immune functions and thus physical health [39, 40]. Studies have tested this conjecture by investigating the association between face evaluations and actual health records [42, 105, 106]. Several pieces of supporting evidence were obtained from these studies. For example, facial masculinity and asymmetry have been linked to actual health status, indexed by antibiotic use and a history of respiratory disease [42]. However, the association between ratings of masculinity and attractiveness and actual health status was modest or absent [105]. Thus, it is possible that sexual dimorphism reflects actual health status, but people are not good at exploiting this information to its full extent, which indicates limited signaling value of sexual dimorphisms. Kalick et al. [106] observed that perceived facial attractiveness mitigated the association between perceived and actual health. More specifically, participants were good at predicting health status based on facial information for moderately attractive faces but not for extremely attractive or unattractive faces. This finding indicates that the signal value of sexual dimorphism was degraded by the halo effect of perceived attractiveness.

Another line of research has directly investigated the association between masculine traits and the strength of the immune response. A comprehensive study [107] on multiple aspects of the immune response, including both humoral and cell-mediated immunity and serum levels of free testosterone, dihydrotestosterone (DHT), and dehydroepiandrosterone, identified a positive association between the strength of the immune response to influenza vaccination and free testosterone and DHT; however, many of the pairwise correlations were null. Another study [40] investigated the association between facial attractiveness, testosterone levels, and immune response to hepatitis B vaccination. The results revealed that males with high testosterone levels showed stronger immune responses, and males with stronger immune responses were rated more attractive by females than those with weak immune responses, giving strong support to the immunocompetence handicap theory. These associations were particularly prominent in males with low glucocorticoid levels. Thus, existing studies provide some support for the immunocompetence handicap theory [39, 40] but at the same time reveal the need for further modification of this theory by integrating multiple measures of immune response and hormonal status.

6. Potential explanations for failure to find signal value of sexually dimorphic features

Many attractiveness perception studies in humans rely on the assumption that attractive features function as signals of, and advertise, the biological quality of an individual to the opposite sex. This assumption has garnered some support from behavioral studies on the human attractiveness perception of faces [46, 66–70] and voices [88–90, 93, 95]. Several of these studies show that people prefer sexually dimorphic traits indicative of high reproductivity [62, 66–70] and immunocompetence [108] and a low level of fluctuating asymmetry that reflects robustness against biological harm [42, 43]. However, it is currently difficult to assume that evolutionary theory of attractive perception has been unanimously supported by empirical studies.

There are several pieces of evidence indicating the association between sexually dimorphic traits, such as low-pitched voice, facial masculinity, and testosterone level [83, 100, 101]. However, there are few studies on the link between these masculine features, actual health records, reproductive prowess indexed by semen quality, and immunocompetence.

The reason for the lack of clear evidence for the signal value of sexual dimorphism is yet to be clarified. One reason, of course, is that the attractiveness of sexual dimorphism, including sexual dimorphism and the neural machinery to perceive sexual dimorphism as attractive, has evolved for reasons other than its signal value. The Fisherian runaway hypothesis [109] proposes that sexually dimorphic features, such as the grandiose ornament of the peacock's tail, can evolve even when they do not signal biological fitness. First, certain features emerge in one sex either as a signal of biological quality or as a result of perceptual bias. If the feature sexually attracts the opposite sex, individuals with this feature achieve greater reproductive success. Thus, this is an adaptive strategy for the other sex to mate with individuals with this feature. Through generations, the development of this feature and preference for it in individuals of the opposite sex reinforce each other in a positive feedback loop with no regard to the actual signal value. In this case, there is only loose or no association between the sexually selected feature and biological quality.

Another reason is that most existing studies have focused on the attractiveness perception of features that reflect biological fitness at the trait level, and a relatively small number of studies have dealt with the attractiveness perception of features that fluctuate within an individual depending on one's physical state [108]. The probability of bearing offspring with "good gene" depends on the mating partner's current health status as well as the baseline level of reproductivity and biological quality. Sexual dimorphism in the face and voice is a stable marker of trait-level biological quality, and current health status is more sensitively reflected in features such as skin texture [110], adiposity [108, 111], and subtle timbral features of jitter and simmer in voice [112]. Several studies have raised the possibility that these state markers are more tightly linked to health status and exert stronger influences on attractiveness perception [108, 110, 111] and mating strategy than features reflecting unchanging trait-level biological fitness. Scott et al. [110] reported that skin coloration is prioritized over facial masculinity in the evaluation of health status and attractiveness from facial information. Likewise, Rantala et al. [108] revealed a stronger association between circulating testosterone and adiposity than between circulating testosterone and masculinity in the face and body. Furthermore, the link between facial attractiveness and the strength of the immune response to hepatitis B vaccination is mediated by adiposity and not by masculinity.

7. Conclusion

Several behavioral studies have found supporting evidence for the assertion that attractive features have been sexually selected; however, this pattern is not necessarily unequivocal. Furthermore, there is limited evidence for a link between sexually dimorphic traits and biological traits, such as immunocompetence and reproductivity. In its current state, existing studies mainly focus on attractiveness perception of phenotypes that are supposed to reflect trait-level fitness and health status. Furthermore, a few studies have incorporated the measurement of multiple hormones, failing to appreciate a potential interaction between sex steroids and other endocrinological factors influencing attractiveness perception. Moreover, as most studies have adopted a correlational design, their ability to identify the causality of the observed associations is limited. More comprehensive studies on the perception of attractiveness, incorporating experimental manipulation of sex-steroid administration, would enrich the knowledge in this field of research and provide a more solid basis to discuss the validity of the evolutionary roots of human attractiveness perception.

Conflict of interest

The author declares no conflict of interest.

Author details

Hirokazu Doi
Department of Information and Management Systems Engineering, Nagaoka University of Technology, Nagaoka City, Niigata Prefecture, Japan

*Address all correspondence to: hdoi_0407@yahoo.co.jp

References

[1] LeDoux JE. Emotion circuits in the brain. Annual Review of Neuroscience. 2000;**2000**(23):155-184

[2] Carr JA. I'll take the low road: The evolutionary underpinnings of visually triggered fear. Frontiers in Neuroscience. 2015;**9**:414. DOI: 10.3389/fnins.2015.00414

[3] Dabbs JM, Carr TS, Frady RL, Riad JK. Testosterone, crime, and misbehavior among 692 male prison inmates. Personality and Individual Differences. 1995;**18**(5):627-633. DOI: 10.1016/0191-8869(94)00177-T

[4] Batrinos ML. Testosterone and aggressive behavior in man. International Journal of Endocrinology Metabolism. 2012;**10**(3):563-568. DOI: 10.5812/ijem.3661

[5] Wu Y, Shen B, Liao J, Li Y, Zilioli S, Li H. Single dose testosterone administration increases impulsivity in the intertemporal choice task among healthy males. Hormones and Behavior. 2020;**118**:104634. DOI: 10.1016/j.yhbeh.2019.104634

[6] Mazur A, Booth A. Testosterone and dominance in men. Behavioral and Brain Sciences. 1998;**21**(3):353-397. DOI: 10.1017/S0140525X98001228

[7] Doi H, Nishitani S, Shinohara K. Sex difference in the relationship between salivary testosterone and inter-temporal choice. Hormones and Behavior. 2015;**69**:50-58. DOI: 10.1016/j.yhbeh.2014.12.005

[8] Doi H, Basadonne I, Venuti P, Shinohara K. Negative correlation between salivary testosterone concentration and preference for sophisticated music in males. Personality and Individual Differences. 2018;**125**:106-111. DOI: 10.1016/j.paid.2017.11.041

[9] Sapienza P, Zingales L, Maestripieri D. Gender differences in financial risk aversion and career choices are affected by testosterone. Proceedings of the National Academy of Sciences of the United States of America. 2009;**106**(36):15268-15273. DOI: 10.1073/pnas.0907352106

[10] Shahani-Denning C. Physical attractiveness bias in hiring: What is beautiful is good. Hofstra Horizons. 2003:15-18

[11] Shahani-Denning C, Dudhat P, Tevet R, Andreoli N. Effect of physical attractiveness on selection decisions in India and the United States. International Journal of Management. 2010;**27**(1):37

[12] Morrow PC, McElroy JC, Stamper BG, Wilson MA. The effects of physical attractiveness and other demographic characteristics on promotion decisions. Journal of Management. 1990;**16**(4):723-736. DOI: 10.1177/014920639001600405

[13] Dion K, Berscheid E, Walster E. What is beautiful is good. Journal of Personality and Social Psychology. 1972;**24**(3):285-290. DOI: 10.1037/h0033731

[14] Batres C, Shiramizu V. Examining the “attractiveness halo effect” across cultures. Current Psychology. 2022

[15] Eagly AH, Ashmore RD, Makhijani MG, Longo LC. What is beautiful is good, but…: A meta-analytic review of research on the physical

attractiveness stereotype. Psychological Bulletin. 1991;**110**(1):109-128. DOI: 10.1037/0033-2909.110.1.109

[16] Rhodes G, Simmons LW, Peters M. Attractiveness and sexual behavior: Does attractiveness enhance mating success? Evolution and Human Behavior. 2005;**26**(2):186-201. DOI: 10.1016/j.evolhumbehav.2004.08.014

[17] Karraker A, Sicinski K, Moynihan D. Your face is your fortune: Does adolescent attractiveness predict intimate relationships later in life? The Journals of Gerontology. Series B, Psychological Sciences and Social Sciences. 2017;**72**(1):187-199. DOI: 10.1093/geronb/gbv112

[18] Lincoln GA. Reproductive seasonality and maturation throughout the complete life-cycle in the mouflon ram (Ovis musimon). Animal Reproduction Science. 1998;**53**(1-4):87-105. DOI: 10.1016/s0378-4320(98)00129-8

[19] Toledano-Díaz A, Santiago-Moreno J, Gómez-Brunet A, Pulido-Pastor A, López-Sebastián A. Horn growth related to testosterone secretion in two wild Mediterranean ruminant species: The Spanish ibex (Capra pyrenaica hispanica) and European mouflon (Ovis orientalis musimon). Animal Reproduction Science. 2007;**102**(3-4):300-307. DOI: 10.1016/j.anireprosci.2006.10.021

[20] Malo AF, Roldan ER, Garde JJ, Soler AJ, Vicente J, Gortazar C, et al. What does testosterone do for red deer males? Proceedings of the Biological Sciences. 2009;**276**(1658):971-980. DOI: 10.1098/rspb.2008.1367

[21] Goldey KL, van Anders SM. Sexual modulation of testosterone: Insights for humans from across species. Adaptive Human Behavior and Physiology. 2015;**1**:93-123

[22] McLachlan RI, Wreford NG, Robertson DM, de Kretser DM. Hormonal control of spermatogenesis. Trends in Endocrinology and Metabolism. 1995;**6**(3):95-101. DOI: 10.1016/1043-2760(94)00215-p

[23] Gervásio CG, Bernuci MP, Silva-de-Sá MF, Rosa-E-Silva AC. The role of androgen hormones in early follicular development. ISRN Obstetrics Gynecology. 2014;**2014**:818010. DOI: 10.1155/2014/818010

[24] Puts DA, Pope LE, Hill AK, Cárdenas RA, Welling LL, Wheatley JR, et al. Fulfilling desire: Evidence for negative feedback between men's testosterone, sociosexual psychology, and sexual partner number. Hormones and Behavior. 2015;**70**:14-21. DOI: 10.1016/j.yhbeh.2015.01.006

[25] Riley A, Riley E. Controlled studies on women presenting with sexual drive disorder: I. Endocrine status. Journal of Sex & Marital Therapy. 2000;**26**(3):269-283. DOI: 10.1080/00926230050084669

[26] Eisenegger C, Naef M, Snozzi R, Heinrichs M, Fehr E. Prejudice and truth about the effect of testosterone on human bargaining behaviour. Nature. 2010;**463**(7279):356-359. DOI: 10.1038/nature08711

[27] Dreher JC, Dunne S, Pazderska A, Frodl T, Nolan JJ, O'Doherty JP. Testosterone causes both prosocial and antisocial status-enhancing behaviors in human males. Proceedings of the National Academy of Sciences of the United States of America. 2016;**113**(41):11633-11638. DOI: 10.1073/pnas.1608085113

[28] Wu Y, Zhang Y, Ou J, Hu Y, Zilioli S. Exogenous testosterone increases the audience effect in healthy males: Evidence for the social status hypothesis.

Proceedings of the Biological Sciences. 1931;**2020**(287):20200976. DOI: 10.1098/rspb.2020.0976

[29] Gettler LT, McDade TW, Feranil AB, Kuzawa CW. Longitudinal evidence that fatherhood decreases testosterone in human males. Proceedings of the National Academy of Sciences of the United States of America. 2011;**108**(39):16194-16199. DOI: 10.1073/pnas.1105403108

[30] Fleming AS, Corter C, Stallings J, Steiner M. Testosterone and prolactin are associated with emotional responses to infant cries in new fathers. Hormones and Behavior. 2002;**42**(4):399-413. DOI: 10.1006/hbeh.2002.1840

[31] Mayr E. Cause and effect in biology. Science. 1961;**134**(3489):1501-1506. DOI: 10.1126/science.134.3489.1501

[32] Nesse RM. Tinbergen's four questions: Two proximate, two evolutionary. Evolution, Medicine, and Public Health. 2018;**2019**(1):2. DOI: 10.1093/emph/eoy035

[33] Kou H, Xie Q, Bi T. Mechanisms for the cognitive processing of attractiveness in adult and infant faces: From the evolutionary perspective. Frontiers in Psychology. 2020;**2020**(11):436. DOI: 10.3389/fpsyg.2020.00436

[34] Zahavi A. The cost of honesty (further remarks on the handicap principle). Journal of Theoretical Biology. 1977;**67**(3):603-605. DOI: 10.1016/0022-5193(77)90061-3

[35] Zahavi A. Mate selection-a selection for a handicap. Journal of Theoretical Biology. 1975;**53**(1):205-214. DOI: 10.1016/0022-5193(75)90111-3

[36] Petrie M, Halliday T, Sanders C. Peahens prefer peacocks with elaborate trains. Animal Behaviour. 1991;**41**:323-331. DOI: 10.1016/S0003-3472(05)80484-1

[37] Pryke SR, Andersson S. Experimental evidence for female choice and energetic costs of male tail elongation in red-collared widowbirds. Biological Journal of the Linnean Society. 2005;**86**:35-43. DOI: 10.1111/J.1095-8312.2005.00522.X

[38] Preston BT, Stevenson IR, Lincoln GA, Monfort SL, Pilkington JG, Wilson K. Testes size, testosterone production and reproductive behaviour in a natural mammalian mating system. The Journal of Animal Ecology. 2012;**81**(1):296-305. DOI: 10.1111/j.1365-2656.2011.01907.x

[39] Folstad I, Karter A. Parasites, Bright males, and the immunocompetence handicap. The American Naturalist. 1992;**139**(3):603-622

[40] Rantala MJ, Moore FR, Skrinda I, Krama T, Kivleniece I, Kecko S, et al. Evidence for the stress-linked immunocompetence handicap hypothesis in humans. Nature Communications. 2012;**3**:694. DOI: 10.1038/ncomms1696

[41] Langlois JH, Roggman LA, Casey RJ, Ritter JM, Rieser-Danner LA, Jenkins VY. Infant preferences for attractive faces: Rudiments of a stereotype? Developmental Psychology. 1987;**23**(3):363-369. DOI: 10.1037/0012-1649.23.3.363

[42] Thornhill R, Gangestad SW. Facial sexual dimorphism, developmental stability, and susceptibility to disease in men and women. Evolution and Human Behavior. 2006;**27**(2):131-144

[43] Gangestad SW, Thornhill R, Yeo RA. Facial attractiveness, developmental stability, and fluctuating asymmetry.

Ethology & Sociobiology. 1994;**15**(2):73-85. DOI: 10.1016/0162-3095(94)90018-3

[44] Swaddle JP, Cuthill IC. Asymmetry and human facial attractiveness: Symmetry may not always be beautiful. Proceedings of the Biological Sciences. 1995;**261**(1360):111-116. DOI: 10.1098/rspb.1995.0124

[45] Lorenz K. Die angeborenen Formen möglicher Erfahrung. Zeitschrift für Tierpsychologie. 1943;**5**:233-519. DOI: 10.1111/j.1439-0310.1943.tb00655.x

[46] Glocker ML, Langleben DD, Ruparel K, Loughead JW, Gur RC, Sachser N. Baby schema in infant faces induces cuteness perception and motivation for caretaking in adults. Ethology. 2009;**115**(3):257-263. DOI: 10.1111/j.1439-0310.2008.01603.x

[47] Glocker ML, Langleben DD, Ruparel K, Loughead JW, Valdez JN, Griffin MD, et al. Baby schema modulates the brain reward system in nulliparous women. Proceedings of the National Academy of Sciences of the United States of America. 2009;**106**(22):9115-9119. DOI: 10.1073/pnas.0811620106

[48] Hahn AC, DeBruine LM, Fisher CI, Jones BC. The reward value of infant facial cuteness tracks within-subject changes in women's salivary testosterone. Hormones and Behavior. 2015;**67**:54-59. DOI: 10.1016/j.yhbeh.2014.11.010

[49] Holtfrerich SK, Schwarz KA, Sprenger C, Reimers L, Diekhof EK. Endogenous testosterone and exogenous oxytocin modulate attentional processing of infant faces. PLoS One. 2016;**11**(11):e0166617. DOI: 10.1371/journal.pone.0166617

[50] Berry DS, Zebrowitz-McArthur L. What's in a face?: Facial maturity and the attribution of legal responsibility. Personality and Social Psychology Bulletin. 1988;**14**(1):23-33. DOI: 10.1177/0146167288141003

[51] Masip J, Garrido E, Herrero C. Facial appearance and impressions of credibility: The effects of facial babyishness and age on person perception. International Journal of Psychology. 2004;**39**(4):276-289. DOI: 10.1080/00207590444000014

[52] Doi H, Morikawa M, Inadomi N, Aikawa K, Uetani M, Shinohara K. Neural correlates of babyish adult face processing in men. Neuropsychologia 2017;**97**:9-17. DOI: 10.1016/j.neuropsychologia.2017.01.017.

[53] Perrett DI, Lee KJ, Penton-Voak I, Rowland D, Yoshikawa S, Burt DM, et al. Effects of sexual dimorphism on facial attractiveness. Nature. 1998;**394**(6696):884-887. DOI: 10.1038/29772

[54] Scott IM, Clark AP, Josephson SC, Boyette AH, Cuthill IC, Fried RL, et al. Human preferences for sexually dimorphic faces may be evolutionarily novel. Proceedings of the National Academy of Sciences of the United States of America. 2014;**111**(40):14388-14393. DOI: 10.1073/pnas.1409643111

[55] Fraccaro PJ, Feinberg DR, DeBruine LM, Little AC, Watkins CD, Jones BC. Correlated male preferences for femininity in female faces and voices. Evolutionary Psychology. 2010;**8**(3):447-461. DOI: 10.1177/147470491000800311

[56] O'Connor JJ, Fraccaro PJ, Pisanski K, Tigue CC, Feinberg DR. Men's preferences for women's femininity in dynamic cross-modal stimuli. PLoS One. 2013;**8**(7):e69531. DOI: 10.1371/journal.pone.0069531

[57] Little AC, Jones BC, Feinberg DR, Perrett DI. Men's strategic preferences for

femininity in female faces. British Journal of Psychology. 2014;**105**(3):364-381. DOI: 10.1111/bjop.12043

[58] Burriss RP, Welling LLM, Puts DA. Men's attractiveness predicts their preference for female facial femininity when judging for short-term, but not long-term, partners. Personality and Individual Differences. 2011;**50**(5):542-546. DOI: 10.1016/j.paid.2010.11.022

[59] Welling LL, Jones BC, DeBruine LM, Smith FG, Feinberg DR, Little AC, et al. Men report stronger attraction to femininity in women's faces when their testosterone levels are high. Hormones and Behavior. 2008;**54**(5):703-708. DOI: 10.1016/j.yhbeh.2008.07.012

[60] Welling LLM, Persola L, Wheatley JR, Cárdenas RA, Puts DA. Competition and men's face preferences. Personality and Individual Differences. 2013;**54**(3):414-419

[61] Losecaat Vermeer AB, Riečanský I, Eisenegger C. Competition, testosterone, and adult neurobehavioral plasticity. Progress in Brain Research. 2016;**229**:213-238. DOI: 10.1016/bs.pbr.2016.05.004

[62] Han C, Zhang Y, Lei X, Li X, Morrison ER, Wu Y. Single dose testosterone administration increases men's facial femininity preference in a Chinese population. Psychoneuroendocrinology. 2020;**115**:-104630. DOI: 10.1016/j.psyneuen.2020.104630

[63] Bird BM, Welling LLM, Ortiz TL, Moreau BJP, Hansen S, Emond M, et al. Effects of exogenous testosterone and mating context on men's preferences for female facial femininity. Hormones and Behavior. 2016;**85**:76-85. DOI: 10.1016/j.yhbeh.2016.08.003

[64] Scott IM, Clark AP, Boothroyd LG, Penton-Voak IS. Do men's faces really signal heritable immunocompetence? Behavioral Ecology. 2013;**24**(3):579-589. DOI: 10.1093/beheco/ars092

[65] Rhodes G. The evolutionary psychology of facial beauty. Annual Review of Psychology. 2006;**57**:199-226. DOI: 10.1146/annurev.psych.57.102904.190208

[66] Roney JR, Simmons ZL. Women's estradiol predicts preference for facial cues of men's testosterone. Hormones and Behavior. 2008;**53**(1):14-19. DOI: 10.1016/j.yhbeh.2007.09.008

[67] Penton-Voak IS, Perrett DI, Castles DL, Kobayashi T, Burt DM, Murray LK, et al. Menstrual cycle alters face preference. Nature. 1999;**399**(6738):741-742. DOI: 10.1038/21557

[68] Penton-Voak IS, Perrett DI. Female preference for male faces changes cyclically: Further evidence. Evolution and Human Behavior. 2000;**21**(1):39-48. DOI: 10.1016/S1090-5138(99)00033-1

[69] Jones BC, Little AC, Boothroyd L, Debruine LM, Feinberg DR, Smith MJ, et al. Commitment to relationships and preferences for femininity and apparent health in faces are strongest on days of the menstrual cycle when progesterone level is high. Hormones and Behavior. 2005;**48**(3):283-290. DOI: 10.1016/j.yhbeh.2005.03.010

[70] Roney JR, Hanson KN, Durante KM, Maestripieri D. Reading men's faces: women's mate attractiveness judgments track men's testosterone and interest in infants. Proceedings of the Biological Sciences. 2006;**273**(1598):2169-2175. DOI: 10.1098/rspb.2006.3569

[71] Marcinkowska UM, Helle S, Jones BC, Jasienska G. Does testosterone predict women's preference for

facial masculinity? PLoS One. 2019;**14**(2):e0210636. DOI: 10.1371/journal.pone.0210636

[72] Jones BC, Hahn AC, Fisher CI, Wang H, Kandrik M, Han C, et al. No compelling evidence that preferences for facial masculinity track changes in Women's hormonal status. Psychological Science. 2018;**29**(6):996-1005. DOI: 10.1177/0956797618760197

[73] Marcinkowska UM, Ellison PT, Galbarczyk A, Milkowska K, Pawlowski B, Thune I, et al. Lack of support for relation between woman's masculinity preference, estradiol level and mating context. Hormones and Behavior. 2016;**78**:1-7. DOI: 10.1016/j.yhbeh.2015.10.012

[74] Alexander GM, Sherwin BB, Bancroft J, Davidson DW. Testosterone and sexual behavior in oral contraceptive users and nonusers: A prospective study. Hormones and Behavior. 1990;**24**(3):388-402. DOI: 10.1016/0018-506x(90)90017-r

[75] Bloch M, Schmidt PJ, Su T-P, Tobin MB, Rubinow DR. Pituitary-adrenal hormones and testosterone across the menstrual cycle in women with premenstrual syndrome and controls. Biological Psychiatry. 1998;**43**(12):897-903. DOI: 10.1016/S0006-3223(98)00403-X

[76] Welling LL, Jones BC, DeBruine LM, Conway CA, Law Smith MJ, Little AC, et al. Raised salivary testosterone in women is associated with increased attraction to masculine faces. Hormones and Behavior. 2007;**52**(2):156-161. DOI: 10.1016/j.yhbeh.2007.01.010

[77] Bobst C, Sauter S, Foppa A, Lobmaier JS. Early follicular testosterone level predicts preference for masculinity in male faces - but not for women taking hormonal contraception. Psychoneuroendocrinology. 2014;**41**:142-150. DOI: 10.1016/j.psyneuen.2013.12.012

[78] Jones BC, Hahn AC, DeBruine LM. Ovulation, sex hormones, and Women's mating psychology. Trends in Cognitive Sciences. 2019;**23**(1):51-62. DOI: 10.1016/j.tics.2018.10.008

[79] Krejza J, Sledziewski R, Tabedzki M, Chen R, Krzystanek E, Arkuszewski M, et al. Faces of men with high serum testosterone are less attractive for women during the fertility phase of the menstrual cycle. bioRxiv. 2021. DOI: 10.1101/2021.07.22.453412

[80] Fitch WT, Giedd J. Morphology and development of the human vocal tract: A study using magnetic resonance imaging. The Journal of the Acoustical Society of America. 1999;**106**(3 Pt 1):1511-1522. DOI: 10.1121/1.427148

[81] Newman SR, Butler J, Hammond EH, Gray SD. Preliminary report on hormone receptors in the human vocal fold. Journal of Voice. 2000;**14**(1):72-81. DOI: 10.1016/s0892-1997(00)80096-x

[82] Puts DA, Hill AK, Bailey DH, Walker RS, Rendall D, Wheatley JR, et al. Sexual selection on male vocal fundamental frequency in humans and other anthropoids. Proceedings of the Biological Sciences. 1829;**2016**(283):20152830. DOI: 10.1098/rspb.2015.2830

[83] Schild C, Aung T, Kordsmeyer TL, Cardenas RA, Puts DA, Penke L. Linking human male vocal parameters to perceptions, body morphology, strength and hormonal profiles in contexts of sexual selection. Scientific Reports. 2020;**10**(1):21296. DOI: 10.1038/s41598-020-77940-z

[84] Feinberg DR, Jones BC, Law Smith MJ, Moore FR, DeBruine LM,

Cornwell RE, et al. Menstrual cycle, trait estrogen level, and masculinity preferences in the human voice. Hormones and Behavior. 2006;**49**(2):215-222. DOI: 10.1016/j.yhbeh.2005.07.004

[85] Fitch WT. Vocal tract length and formant frequency dispersion correlate with body size in rhesus macaques. The Journal of the Acoustical Society of America. 1997;**102**(2 Pt 1):1213-1222. DOI: 10.1121/1.421048

[86] González J. Formant frequencies and body size of speaker: A weak relationship in adult humans. Journal of Phonetics. 2004;**32**:277-287

[87] Puts DA, Hodges CR, Cárdenas RA, Gaulin SJC. Men's voices as dominance signals: Vocal fundamental and formant frequencies influence dominance attributions among men. Evolution and Human Behavior. 2007;**28**(5):340-344

[88] Collins SA. Men's voices and women's choices. Animal Behaviour. 2000;**60**(6):773-780. DOI: 10.1006/anbe.2000.1523

[89] Feinberg DR, Jones BC, Little AC, Burt DM, Perrett DI. Manipulations of fundamental and formant frequencies influence the attractiveness of human male voices. Animal Behaviour. 2005;**69**(3):561-568. DOI: 10.1016/j.anbehav.2004.06.012

[90] Collins SA, Missing C. Vocal and visual attractiveness are related in women. Animal Behaviour. 2003;**65**(5):997-1004. DOI: 10.1006/anbe.2003.2123

[91] Xu Y, Lee A, Wu WL, Liu X, Birkholz P. Human vocal attractiveness as signaled by body size projection. PLoS One. 2013;**8**(4):e62397. DOI: 10.1371/journal.pone.0062397

[92] Bruckert L, Liénard JS, Lacroix A, Kreutzer M, Leboucher G. Women use voice parameters to assess men's characteristics. Proceedings of the Biological Sciences. 2006;**273**(1582):83-89. DOI: 10.1098/rspb.2005.3265

[93] Sell A, Bryant GA, Cosmides L, Tooby J, Sznycer D, von Rueden C, et al. Adaptations in humans for assessing physical strength from the voice. Proceedings of the Biological Sciences. 2010;**277**(1699):3509-3518. DOI: 10.1098/rspb.2010.0769

[94] Little AC, Connely J, Feinberg DR, Jones BC, Roberts SC. Human preference for masculinity differs according to context in faces, bodies, voices, and smell. Behavioral Ecology. 2011;**22**(4):862-868. DOI: 10.1093/beheco/arr061

[95] Apicella CL, Feinberg DR, Marlowe FW. Voice pitch predicts reproductive success in male hunter-gatherers. Biology Letters. 2007;**3**(6):682-684. DOI: 10.1098/rsbl.2007.0410

[96] Puts DA. Cyclic variation in women's preferences for masculine traits : Potential hormonal causes. Human Nature. 2006;**17**(1):114-127. DOI: 10.1007/s12110-006-1023-x

[97] Pisanski K, Hahn AC, Fisher CI, DeBruine LM, Feinberg DR, Jones BC. Changes in salivary estradiol predict changes in women's preferences for vocal masculinity. Hormones and Behavior. 2014;**66**(3):493-497. DOI: 10.1016/j.yhbeh.2014.07.006

[98] Kandrik M, Hahn AC, Wincenciak J, Fisher CI, Pisanski K, Feinberg DR, et al. Are Men's perceptions of sexually dimorphic vocal characteristics related to their testosterone levels? PLoS One. 2016;**11**(11):e0166855. DOI: 10.1371/journal.pone.0166855

[99] Riggs BL, Khosla S, Melton LJ 3rd. Sex steroids and the construction and conservation of the adult skeleton. Endocrine Reviews. 2002;**23**(3):279-302. DOI: 10.1210/edrv.23.3.0465

[100] Penton-Voak IS, Chen JY. High salivary testosterone is linked to masculine male facial appearance in humans. Evolution and Human Behavior. 2004;**25**(4):229-241

[101] Dabbs JM Jr, Mallinger A. High testosterone levels predict low voice pitch among men. Personality and Individual Differences. 1999;**27**(4):801-804. DOI: 10.1016/S0191-8869(98)00272-4

[102] Soler C, Núñez M, Gutiérrez R, Núñez J, Medina P, Sancho M, et al. Facial attractiveness in men provides clues to semen quality. Evolution and Human Behavior. 2003;**24**(3):199-207. DOI: 10.1016/S1090-5138(03)00013-8

[103] Peters M, Rhodes G, Simmons LW. Does attractiveness in men provide clues to semen quality? Journal of Evolutionary Biology. 2008;**21**(2):572-579. DOI: 10.1111/j.1420-9101.2007.01477.x

[104] Simmons LW, Peters M, Rhodes G. Low pitched voices are perceived as masculine and attractive but do they predict semen quality in men? PLoS One. 2011;**6**(12):e29271. DOI: 10.1371/journal.pone.0029271

[105] Rhodes G, Chan J, Zebrowitz LA, Simmons LW. Does sexual dimorphism in human faces signal health? Proceedings of the Biological Sciences. 2003;**270**(Suppl 1):S93-S95. DOI: 10.1098/rsbl.2003.0023

[106] Kalick SM, Zebrowitz LA, Langlois JH, Johnson RM. Does human facial attractiveness honestly advertise health? Longitudinal data on an evolutionary question. Psychological Science. 1998;**9**(1):8-13

[107] Nowak J, Pawłowski B, Borkowska B, Augustyniak D, Drulis-Kawa Z. No evidence for the immunocompetence handicap hypothesis in male humans. Scientific Reports. 2018;**8**(1):7392. DOI: 10.1038/s41598-018-25694-0

[108] Rantala MJ, Coetzee V, Moore FR, Skrinda I, Kecko S, Krama T, et al. Adiposity, compared with masculinity, serves as a more valid cue to immunocompetence in human mate choice. Proceedings of the Biological Sciences. 2013;**280**(1751):20122495. DOI: 10.1098/rspb.2012.2495

[109] Fisher RA. The evolution of sexual preference. The Eugenics Review. 1915;**7**(3):184-192

[110] Stephen ID, Scott IML, Coetzee V, Pound N, Perrett DI, Penton-Voak IS. Cross-cultural effects of color, but not morphological masculinity, on perceived attractiveness of men's faces. Evolution and Human Behavior. 2012;**33**(4):260-267

[111] de Jager S, Coetzee N, Coetzee V. Facial adiposity, attractiveness, and health: A review. Frontiers in Psychology. 2018;**9**:2562. DOI: 10.3389/fpsyg.2018.02562

[112] Asiaee M, Vahedian-Azimi A, Atashi SS, Keramatfar A, Nourbakhsh M. Voice quality evaluation in patients with COVID-19: An acoustic analysis. Journal of Voice. 2020;**S0892-1997**(20):30368-30364. DOI: 10.1016/j.jvoice.2020.09.024

Section 3

Deficiencies and Substitution of Testosterone

Chapter 5

Lung Health and Hypoandrogenism

Nidia N. Gomez, Verónica S. Biaggio, Eloy Salinas, Silvana N. Piguillem, María Eugenia Ciminari, María Verónica Pérez Chaca and Silvina Mónica Álvarez

Abstract

Epidemiological reports offer evidence that gender differences mediate respiratory diseases. Male sex is a major risk factor for respiratory distress syndrome and bronchopulmonary dysplasia in neonates. An imbalance between oxidants/antioxidants leads to stress, which has been implicated in airway disease development. It is known that androgens deficiency induces oxidative stress and lipid peroxidation in the lung, synchronically with changes in the expression of cytoprotective markers. Additionally, males are more susceptible to acute and chronic inflammation after toxicant exposure. Besides, nutrition is an important factor, given that lipids are the main blocks for surfactant production and for testosterone synthesis. Also, an adequate amount of Zn in the diet prevents inflammation and is necessary for testosterone and androgen receptor structure and function. This chapter focuses on understanding the effect and clinical implications of testosterone deficiency on lung tissue as well as exploring the role of lipids and zinc in the outcome of several respiratory diseases.

Keywords: androgens, lung, male, inflammation, respiratory diseases

1. Introduction

1.1 Lung structure and sex differences

Biological sex mediates differences in lung disease incidence and pathophysiology, which emerge from sex variations in lung structure and function itself and also in the lung immune cells that are recruited during inflammation [1]. In healthy women, large conducting airways are 30% smaller than in healthy men and sex variations in the airway luminal area persist even after matching for lung size. Larger conducting airways are the main site of airway resistance, linking anatomy to analyzed sex differences in pulmonary physiology [2]. The female lung during intrauterine development has several structural advantages over the male lung. Even if surfactant is produced earlier, the female lung is smaller whereas it has a larger amount of alveoli per unit area. Lung maturation, therefore, is faster in females than in male fetuses. Also, neonatal females have higher expiratory flow rates than males. Regarding respiratory distress syndrome development, bronchopulmonary dysplasia in neonates, and asthma, males present superior risk factors than women during childhood [3].

IntechOpen

In this chapter, we also review sex differences in the structure and function of healthy lungs as well as lungs in pathological conditions that depend on the sex hormones' action. Testosterone deficiency (TD) is very common in older men and is related to different signs and symptoms, such as diminished libido, reduced sexual function, and decreased mobility and energy; which could greatly affect the aging process and quality of life [4, 5]. Androgen receptor (AR) is the intermediary of testosterone effects which is subjected to its sensitivity [6].

Several studies support interdependent sex and endogenous sex hormones effects on lung growth and airways responsiveness that might explain asthma status from puberty to middle age. Puberty is a dynamic process regulated by hormonal signals from the central nervous system that results in sexual maturation. Assessment of the pubertal stage development is different in boys from girls. In boys, androgen production gradually increases both from the testes producing testosterone and from the adrenal glands producing weaker androgens—ultimately leading to puberty. Girls experience increases in estrogen production from the ovaries (driving thelarche and ultimately menarche) and androgens such as androstenedione and DHEA-S from the adrenal glands (driving puberty). In children, pubertal maturation and asthma status may also be affected by corticosteroid treatments [7]. Androgen surge during puberty is capable of conferring protective influences on lung growth in both males and females whereas estrogens could well have deleterious effects in females extending into adult development.

2. Androgen receptor

The androgen receptor (AR) belongs to the steroid and nuclear receptor superfamily. Among this large family of proteins, only five vertebrate steroid receptors are known: androgen, estrogen, progesterone, glucocorticoid, and mineralocorticoid receptors [8–10]. Two subtypes of estrogen receptors have been identified: α and β. Like other steroid receptors, AR is a soluble protein that operates as an intracellular transcriptional factor. AR function is regulated by androgen binding, which initiates sequential conformational receptor changes that affect both receptor-protein and DNA interactions. AR-regulated gene expression is reliable for male sexual differentiation and pubertal changes. The known AR ligands can be classified as steroidal or non-steroidal based on their structure either as agonist or antagonist, based on their ability to activate or inhibit target genes' transcription [8, 9]. AR is mainly expressed in androgen target tissues, such as the prostate, skeletal muscle, liver, lung, and central nervous system (CNS). The highest expression levels are observed in the prostate, adrenal gland, and epididymis as determined by real-time polymerase chain reaction (PCR). AR can be activated by endogenous androgens merging, including testosterone and 5R-dihydrotestosterone (5R-DHT).

Physiologically, functional AR is reliable for male sexual distinction in the uterus and for male pubertal changes. In adult males, androgen is mainly responsible for maintaining libido, spermatogenesis, muscle mass and force, bone mineral density, and also erythropoiesis. Androgens are regularly dispersed all over the entire organism, especially in the lungs.

3. Immune system

Many immune cells in the lungs express ARs and are susceptible to androgens, like ARs on myeloid immune cells (monocytes and macrophages) as they are associated with healthiness and illness. Particularly, we point out androgen influences on lung diseases, such as asthma, chronic obstructive pulmonary disease (COPD), and lung fibrosis.

Immune response differs between males and females because its type and magnitude are influenced by biological sex and age. Genetic (chromosomal) sex differences and those mediated by the action of sex hormones engendered sex differences in the immune system function. Female hormones, mainly estrogens, have been well studied in their numerous functions, while androgen as modulators of the immune system has not been investigated so extensively [8, 9].

Myeloid cell response in the lung is modulated by androgens, which results in the outcome of different lung diseases. Incidence and pathophysiology of lung diseases are mediated by biological sex. These variations emerge from sex differences in the lung structure and function, and also in the immune cells that populate the lung and are recruited to it during inflammation. Before birth, the female lung has several structural advantages over the male lung, as stated in the first paragraph.

Despite lung contribution to structural dissimilarities between the sexes, those differences in lung function and diseases are also influenced by sex hormones. Testosterone and estrogen affect lung macrophage functions [11]; therefore, this may contribute to particular lung disease development. The amount of AR cellular expression and hormone concentration regulates testosterone's immunoregulatory characteristics.

In fact, when we refer to the physiological function of the lung, alveolar macrophages (AM) are the most abundant cell type of the immune system and one of the first cells in contact with the allergenic stimulus. During the inflammatory process, Th2 immune response polarizes AM to an M2 phenotype [12] and the accumulation of M2-polarized AM in the lung correlates with asthma severity [13]. AM (M2) secretes cytokines that recruit eosinophils during allergic lung inflammation [14].

Keselman et al. [15] analyzed the effect of estrogen on macrophage polarization, suggesting an enhanced M2 polarization, which indicates a long-lasting effect on lung inflammation. On the other side, Becerra Diaz et al. [11] evaluated the role of androgens in lung inflammation, particularly AM polarization in allergic lung inflammation, finding out that AM1 expression was restored to control values with androgen-replacement therapy. Both experiments contribute to explaining the sex differences observed in asthma.

4. Surfactant

Pneumocytes are alveolar cells found on the alveoli surface in the lungs. There are two types of cells that cover the alveoli: type I and type II pneumocytes (PTI and PTII, respectively). They are present in a ratio of 1:2. PTI cells form the majority of the epithelium while PTII cells account for only about 15% of peripheral lung cells [16]. Type I pneumocytes are thin squamous cells that cover almost 95% of the alveolar surface. Pneumocytes are connected to each other by tight junctions. The adjacent PTI cells are connected by tight or occluding junctions that prevent leakage of fluid into the alveolar space. During inspiration and expiration, the flat extensions overlap each other. The type I cells are involved in the gaseous exchange between the alveoli and capillaries.

Type II pneumocytes are cubic in shape and they are characterized by microvilli on their surface. The major functions of the type II cells include the secretion of surfactant to reduce surface tension. PTII can convert into PTI cells and regenerate the alveolar surface at the time of injury. The coating of these lipids in alveoli is relevant, without which the alveoli may collapse. The surfactant is secreted by secretory granules called lamellar bodies. These tension active are made up of 70–80% of phospholipids and small proteins called surfactant proteins (sp). Surfactant proteins start to be secreted at about 25 weeks of gestation.

Surfactant is produced in fetal life, and, glucocorticoid receptor (GR) is essential in promoting differentiation and maturation of PTII cells during embryonic life [9, 10, 17]. Antenatal glucocorticoid administration accelerates lung maturation in infants at risk of preterm delivery, largely through increased surfactant protein expression.

Ojeda et al. have shown that testosterone absence alters surfactant phospholipid composition, mainly increasing phosphatidylcholine content [18], and leading to damage in the lung parenchyma. Thus, the male sex is a major risk factor for the development of respiratory distress syndrome, bronchopulmonary dysplasia in neonates [9, 10, 17, 18], and asthma in childhood [9, 17]. Androgen receptor (AR) mediates the effects of male sex steroids in a variety of reproductive and non-reproductive tissues both in males and females under physiological and pathophysiological conditions [9, 10, 17, 18].

5. Androgen deficiency and oxidative stress

It is known that redox balance is important in the airways because it is the first contact with environmental contaminants, particles, cigarette smoke (CS), and pathogens.

Chemically, oxidation is a reaction where a substance loses electrons and is oxidized, which can occur by mechanisms that enhance the production of free radicals (unstable substances with unpaired electrons), developing chain reactions. These reactions are uncontrollable as long as they have sufficient substrate to continue developing and can cause damage to the different components of the cells, especially those of a lipid nature. Antioxidants end the reaction by interacting with intermediate compounds and preventing their spread [19].

Therefore, an imbalance between oxidants/antioxidants induces stress, which has been implicated in the development of airway diseases. Several antioxidant enzymes are critical for maintaining cellular homeostasis and preventing cellular damage [20].

Oxidative stress causes an imbalance in the production of reactive oxygen species (ROS) and reactive nitrogen species (RNS) and their relationship with the antioxidant defense system of lung cells [21]. Some ROS and RNS responsible for oxidative stress such as superoxide, ozone, hydrogen peroxide, hydroxyl radical, nitrate, nitrosyl, and nitrosothiol [22] are produced as by-products of metabolic processes in cells [23] and play a vital role in regulating various biological phenomena, some of which are associated with proinflammatory processes [24].

ROS have a dual involvement in the cell, taking part in different cellular functions, such as defense against infectious agents and signaling systems. On the contrary, its accumulation in biological systems produces oxidative stress, representing an alteration in the pro-oxidant/antioxidant balance, with the ability to oxidize biomolecules (lipids, proteins, DNA), and inhibit their normal structure and function.

One of the indicators of oxidative damage in the lung is lipid peroxidation which causes a considerable amount of DNA-malondialdehyde (MDA) adducts [25]. Lipid peroxidation affects all cell membranes inducing numerous injuries and loss of functions. On the other hand, ferroptosis is a form of cell death characterized by iron-dependent lipid peroxidation, which induces cell death. During ferroptosis, an accumulation of polyunsaturated fatty acids (PUFAs) occurs. This involves PUFA-driven lipid peroxidation that increases cell membrane permeability making the cell more sensitive to oxidation [26]. Enzymatic antioxidants and non-enzymatic antioxidants act together to detoxify the effects of oxidative stress and lipid peroxidation. This synergistic action can be measured using total antioxidant capacity (TAC) [27].

Additionally, males are susceptible to acute neutrophilic inflammation after a single exposure to toxicants, as well as chronic monocytic inflammation after repeated exposures to them. Exposure to ozone has numerous negative effects on lung health and innate pulmonary host defense. Sex differences in lung histology and BAL measurements of lung injury and inflammation were found. Females showed increased damage compared to males, and the expression of inflammatory mediators also varied with sex under basal conditions and following exposure to ozone. This situation indicated a potential sexual dimorphism in the mechanisms associated with the inflammatory response to this air pollutant. Understanding how differentially expressed genes regulate the response to environmental insults may provide the bases to identify sex-specific targets for therapy against acute lung inflammation and injury [28].

There is abundant evidence revealing the action of heat shock proteins (HSPs), mainly in inflammatory conditions. At 30 days after castration, we have shown [20] an increase in oxidative stress markers such as TBARS and antioxidant enzymes expression such as glutathione peroxidase (GPx). During the period of testosterone supplementation, the expression of cytoprotective markers as HSP70i increased, compared to the control group. Additionally, we have observed a decreased HSP27 expression in the testosterone-deprived group. This situation suggests an absence or decrease in cytoprotective properties, which would correlate with the increased level of TBARS found in the lung.

On the other hand, it has been found that a higher expression of Hsp70 reduces the production of nitric oxide (NO) [29], so the higher immunostaining of HSP70 would explain the absence of variations in the concentration of NO in BAL of castrated rats. Therefore, the expression of these proteins would probably play a protective role against androgen deficiency [20].

Besides, sexual hormones play an important role in airway-related diseases and the immune response, leading to pulmonary injuries [30]. Several studies have shown that sex hormones can affect airway tone and inflammation, and exert effects on different lung cell types, including airway smooth muscle [31] and immune cells. These include lung macrophages, neutrophils, dendritic cells, and eosinophils [32, 33].

Testosterone deficiency is commonly observed in male patients with COPD, which is characterized by chronic inflammation of the airways and pulmonary emphysema [34]. As it was previously mentioned, testosterone affects lung macrophage function and this may contribute to the outcome of particular lung diseases. Low levels of endogenous testosterone have been found in men suffering from pathologies such as asthma, COPD, or tuberculosis.

In experimental situations, when testosterone was administered in castrated rats, oxidative stress parameters were modified. For example, TBARS, catalase (CAT), and GPx activities went back to normal values. The same happened with NADPH oxidase (NOX) and GPx expression which were increased in castrated rats and showed a decrease to control values in rats supplemented with testosterone [20, 35].

Epigenetic events cause hyper-methylation (via the promoter) of GSTP1 and Nrf2, which reduces their expression and severely decreases cellular antioxidant capacity. The excessive production of ROS, due to metabolic alterations, and/or extrinsic environmental factors such as pulmonary inflammation along with androgen receptor activation favor oxidative stress state [36]. It is important to highlight that oxidative stress can modify the activity of nuclear and mitochondrial DNA, generating hyper-methylation and mutations [24].

COPD is associated with an abnormal inflammatory response of the airways, alveoli, and microvasculature. Testosterone deficiency also exacerbates COPD symptoms through direct impact on respiratory muscles or decrease exercise capacity. The main cause of the inflammatory process is cigarette smoke [37]. The inflammatory response in COPD progression involves both innate and adaptive immunity [38], which are mediated by multiple immune cell types, including macrophages, T cells, B cells, and neutrophils, as well as epithelial cells [39]. The insufficient control of inflammatory responses to tissue damaging in COPD may be liked to low testosterone.

Overactive tissue and wound healing responses dysregulation in the lung could be used to describe the Th2 response in allergic asthma [3]. Allergic asthma is a chronic disease, which occurs with an altered inflammatory immune response. In the alveolar space of normal lungs, alveolar macrophages are the most abundant immune cells and are the first to come into contact with allergic stimuli. In allergic asthma, Th2 polarizes AM to the M2 phenotype, and the increase of this phenotype is directly related to the severity of pathology. Androgens increase the polarization of AM to M2, although they suppress all other effects of allergic inflammation. These results underscore a little-known role of androgens as modulators of the immune response [3].

Airway epithelial cells are activated to produce inflammatory mediators, including tumor necrosis factor-α (TNF-α), interleukin-1β (IL-1β), granulocyte-macrophage colony-stimulating factor, interleukin-8 (IL-8), and interleukin-6 (IL-6). Nuclear factor kβ (NF-kβ) is crucial for inflammatory pathologies, regulating the transcription of the cytokines TNF-α, IL-1b, and IL-6 [40]. Moreover, androgen deficiency increases inflammation by increasing levels of IL-6, TNF-α, and C-reactive protein [40, 41]. Wang and colleagues [40] found that male castration increased both inflammatory cell recruitment and TNF-α and IL-6 expression. Similar results were found in clinical reports, where higher levels of IL-6, IL-1b, and TNF-α in men with low testosterone levels (hypogonadism) were found [40–42].

In many cases, impaired testicular function and subfertility are associated with obesity, which is a chronic disease associated with metabolic disorders and comorbidity. In this situation, the production of ROS and the release of hormones can affect the hypothalamus-pituitary-testicle axis. Androgen deficiency could further accelerate the increase in adipose tissue and induce a vicious cycle. In individuals where adipose tissue dysfunction and male hypogonadism occur together, a multifactorial pathology of difficult resolution are produced at the pulmonary level [42].

6. Zn deficiency and testosterone

In 1992, Hunt et al. showed that Zn depletion induced a decrease in serum testosterone concentrations in men. Hamdi et al. (1997) also showed a direct action of Zn on testicular steroidogenesis, supporting the idea that Zn deficiency induced hypogonadism mainly from changes in testicular steroidogenesis or indirectly from Leydig cell failure [43, 44].

Omu et al. [45] proved Zn deficiency to be associated with impaired spermatogenesis due to reduced testosterone production, increased oxidative stress, and apoptosis. They showed an obvious reduction of testicular volume, together with increased apoptosis of the testicular cell population. It is known that the zinc transporter (ZnT) family, SLC30a, is involved in the maintenance of Zn homeostasis and in mediating intracellular signaling events.

Zn deficiency has been demonstrated to cause Leydig cells to appear smaller and show endoplasmic reticulum abnormalities when examined under an electron microscope [46, 47]. Chu et al. [48] showed that Zn-deficient (ZnD) Leydig cells were capable of taking up cholesterol and neutral lipids, which are the precursors of sex steroids; however, they could not convert them into sex steroids, thus leading to fertilization impairment due to spermatogenesis arrest.

Two Zn-transporter families regulate Zn homeostasis: Zrt- and Irt-like proteins (ZIPs; SLC39a) and another Zn transporter (ZnT) proteins (SLC30a). ZIPs are responsible for the influx of Zn into the cytoplasm from the cell exterior or from intracellular compartments whereas ZnTs are responsible for Zn efflux to the cells outside or to intracellular organelles [48].

Chu et al. [48] were the first to demonstrate that Znt7 is involved in testosterone synthesis in the mouse testis. The mechanism underlying this process may involve the modulation of the expression levels of testosterone-related factors as well as the expression of the enzymes involved in testosterone synthesis.

On the other hand, according to the crystal structure of the AR DNA binding domain (DBD), each DBD monomer has a core composed of two zinc fingers, each of which consists of four cysteine residues that coordinate a zinc ion. AR, just like other steroid receptors, works as a dimer that binds to the respective response element in the DNA promoter consisting of two equal sites: hexamers sites (5′-AGAACA-3′) separated by a 3 base-pair spacer (IR3). Therefore, this could be another site that could be affected by Zn deficiency, leading to different diseases or deficiencies [49].

Furthermore, in our laboratory we have studied the effect of Zn deficiency in the lung, finding that it induces nitrosative and oxidative stress together with inflammation and alteration in the expression of matrix extracellular proteins [50]. It also increases the expression of apoptosis markers such as Bax and Bad, suggesting that together with the reduced levels of testosterone induced by the same Zn deficiency, the impact on the lung and the risk for chronic and aggressive diseases could be much higher.

7. COVID and testosterone

It has been shown that male individuals are more susceptible to the infection of SARS-CoV-2 than females, and have a higher death rate regardless of age [51].

The explanation for this finding could be: (a) androgens per se are poorly protective over the immune response in males, whereas estrogens (and progesterone) can provide adequate protection to females, stimulating the humoral response to viral infections [52] as a consequence, T levels could not elicit an effective counteracting response to the inflammatory and immunological outcome resulting from a viral infection; (b) a background condition of chronic low T levels—which is estimated to characterize up to 20% of middle-aged/elderly men—may facilitate overall greater incidence and higher severity in men compared to women; and (c) SARS-CoV-2 needs androgen-regulated proteins to invade host cells, including TMPRSS2 for S priming and ACE2 for viral entry, which is expressed in multiple tissues [53].

8. Lung cancer

Lung cancer is the most diagnosed cancer worldwide. Sex hormone concentrations decline as men age, together with increased cancer incidence. For instance, T, DHT, and estrogen (E) were measured in community-dwelling older men and the results revealed that higher levels of androgen were associated with elevated frequency of lung cancer, while they are not associated with the incidence of prostate and colorectal cancer [58]. Therefore, sex hormones may play a role in lung cancer pathophysiology and patient development even if it is not considered as a hormone-sensitive malignancy. An interesting study performed in Canada [59], using a retrospective cohort design, provides further evidence that sex hormones may play a role in lung cancer pathophysiology, and that androgens in particular may have a greater role than previously thought. Male patients, after they were diagnosed with lung cancer, were exposed to androgen pathway manipulation (APM) where most of them received 5-alpha reductase inhibitors and they significantly had better survival when compared to the not exposed ones. Thus, APM utilization in specific lung cancer populations has the potential to be a simple, widely available, and cost-effective treatment for this disease.

It is important to remember that there are two types of lung cancer, non-small cell lung carcinoma (NSCLC) and small cell lung carcinoma, which correspond to 85 and 15% of all lung cancer, respectively. Regarding NSCLC, it is classified into three types: adenocarcinoma, squamous-cell carcinoma, and large-cell carcinoma [54]. The most common is adenocarcinoma that arises from small epithelial type II alveolar cells that produce mucus among other substances [55]. It usually occurs in the lung periphery. When compared to other lung cancers, adenocarcinoma is a slow grower and is usually found before spreading outside the lungs. Squamous-cell carcinoma emerges from early versions of squamous cells from airway epithelial cells in the bronchial tubes in the lungs center.

Large cell carcinoma accounts for 5–10% of lung cancers. This cancer does not show evidence of squamous or glandular maturation therefore it is usually diagnosed by default, excluding other possibilities. It often begins in the central part of the lungs, nearby lymph nodes and into the chest wall [56]. This kind of cancer and tumors are strongly associated with smoking [57].

Female patients generally show better survival rates at any stage of the disease. Histological subtypes of the disease in women include proportionally more adenocarcinoma and less squamous cell carcinoma than in men. Apparently, men have a higher rate of fatal outcomes in lung cancer, but surprisingly, they tend to be less vulnerable to tobacco than women.

9. The analysis of biomarkers

Nowadays, novel therapeutic approaches for the management or monitoring of different lung illnesses are needed. The use of biomarkers and the measurement of their levels as a control for the risk and disease prognosis are considered an encouraging approach. Many types of biomarkers have been identified, which include blood protein biomarkers, cellular biomarkers, and protease enzymes. They have been isolated from different biological sources including sputum, bronchoalveolar fluid, exhaled air, and blood. Sputum samples from patients have been proposed as easily obtained samples that allow complementary diagnostic techniques or alternatives to PCR.

By real-time PCR, reactive oxygen species can be diagnosed from fresh sputum. ROS in sputum could be employed to monitor patients with pathologies such as asthma and COPD. Other modern bioanalytical techniques detect levels of ROS and were used during the COVID-19 pandemic to show oxidative status, at all times [58–61].

Also, higher plasma androgens, particularly DHT, would represent a potential biomarker for lung cancer incidence in older men.

10. Conclusion

We have shown that considerable advances have been made in the understanding of the pathophysiology of lung diseases. It is obvious that the absence of androgens

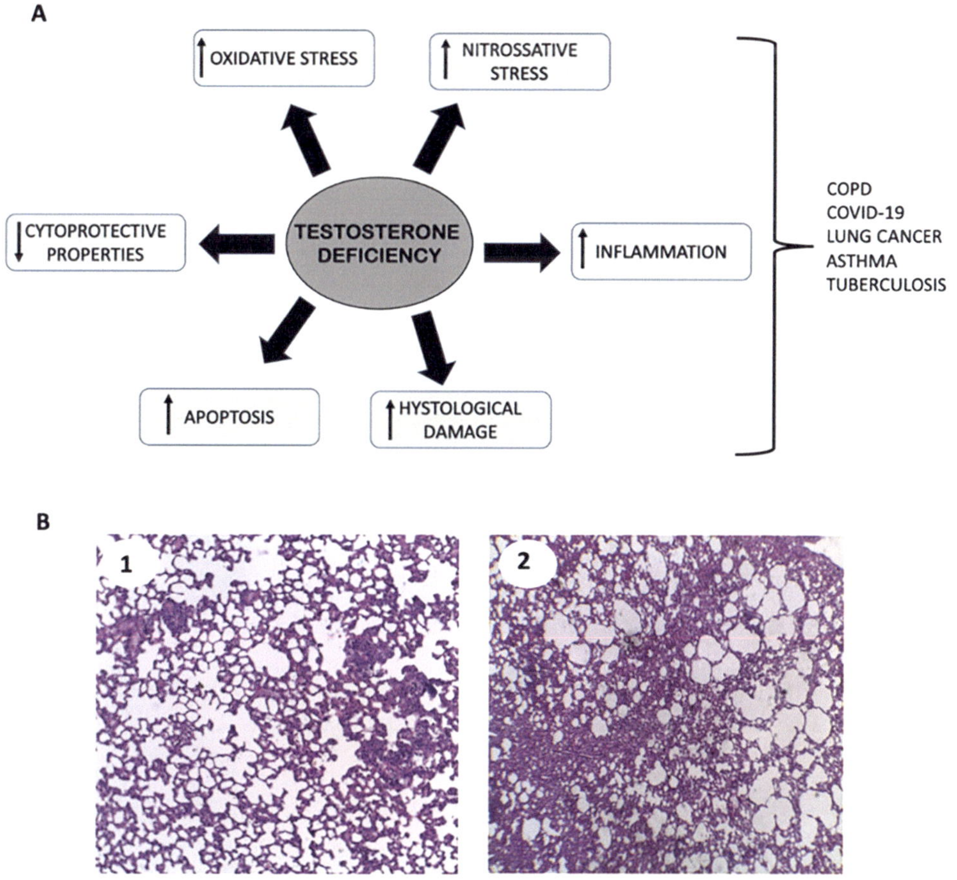

Figure 1.
The different cell functions altered by testosterone deficiency (A). There is an increase in oxidative stress due mainly to a decreased function of antioxidant enzymes. Nitrosative stress is also increased, due to the increased production of NO by iNOS. Inflammation under testosterone deficiency induces a Th1 response. This also induces a decrease in cytoprotective markers, ending in increased apoptosis. Taking together all these effects induces severe histological damage in the lung, making it weaker and more susceptible to diseases, which could end up in COPD, severe prognosis in COVID-19; lung cancer, asthma, and tuberculosis. The histological damage induced by the absence of testosterone after 1 month of treatment (B). (1) Control rat lung. The lung tissue appears normal and the alveoli are homogeneously distributed. The interalveolar septa show typical development of the normal lung. (2) Surgically castrated rat lung. The pulmonary parenchyma presents numerous large spaces caused by the rupture of the interalveolar septa. In other regions, the fibrous connective tissue has increased.

induces oxidative stress and lipid peroxidation in the lung, together with changes in the expression of cytoprotective markers, leading to important alterations in the histoarchitecture of this organ (**Figure 1**). This would lead to a weaker lung, susceptible to undergo several respiratory diseases.

The fact that testosterone levels decrease in elderly men explains the high prevalence of these diseases when compared to women of the same age. All these should be considered to better understand the etiology of respiratory diseases and propose therapies for these patients.

Author details

Nidia N. Gomez[1,2*], Verónica S. Biaggio[1,2], Eloy Salinas[3], Silvana N. Piguillem[1], María Eugenia Ciminari[1], María Verónica Pérez Chaca[1] and Silvina Mónica Álvarez[1,2]

1 Faculty of Chemistry, Department of Biochemistry, Biochemistry and Pharmacy, National University of San Luis, San Luis, Argentina

2 IMIBIO-CONICET, San Luis, Argentina

3 Faculty of Chemistry, Department of Biological Sciences, Biochemistry and Pharmacy, National University of San Luis, San Luis, Argentina

*Address all correspondence to: gomez.nidia@gmail.com

References

[1] Sellau J, Groneberg M, Lotter H. Androgen-dependent immune modulation in parasitic infection. Seminars in Immunopathology. 2019;**41**:213-224. DOI: 10.1007/s00281-018-0722-9

[2] Dominelli PB, Ripoll JG, Cross TJ, Baker SE, Wiggins CHC, Welch BT, et al. Sex differences in large conducting airway anatomy. Journal of Applied Physiology. 2018;**125**:960-965. DOI: 10.1152/japplphysiol.00440.2018

[3] Becerra-Diaz M, Song M, Heller N. Androgen and androgen receptors as regulators of monocyte and macrophage biology in the healthy and diseased lung. Frontiers in Immunology. 2020;**11**:1698. DOI: 10.3389/fimmu.2020.01698

[4] Baum MJ. Sexual differentiation of pheromone processing: Links to male-typical mating behavior and partner preference. Hormones and Behavior, 2009 55: 579-588. https://doi.org/10.1016/j.yhbeh.2009.02.008

[5] Hackett G. An update on the role of testosterone replacement therapy in the management of hypogonadism. Therapeutic Advances in Urology. 2016;**8**(2):147-160. DOI: 10.1177/1756287215617648

[6] Simanainen U, Brogley M, Gao YR, Jimenez M, Harwood DT, Handelsman DJ, et al. Length of the human androgen receptor glutamine tract determines androgen sensitivity in vivo. Molecular and Cellular Endocrinology. 2011;**342**(1-2):81-86. DOI: 10.1016/j.mce.2011.05.011

[7] Zein JG, McManus JM, Sharifi N, Erzurum SC, Marozkina N, Lahm T, et al. Benefits of airway androgen receptor expression in human asthma. American Journal of Respiratory and Critical Care Medicine. 2021;**204**(3):285-293. DOI: 10.1164/rccm.202009-3720OC

[8] Levin ER. Integration of the extra-nuclear and nuclear actions of estrogen. Molecular Endocrinology. 2005;**19**:1951-1959

[9] Stabile L, Davis A, Gubish C, Hopkins T, Luketich JD, Christie N, et al. Human non-small cell lung tumors and cells derived from normal lung express both estrogen receptor and show biological responses to estrogen. Cancer Research. 2002;**62**:2141-2150

[10] Pedram A, Razandi M, Sainson RCA, Kim JK, Hughes CC, Levin ER. A conserved mechanism for steroid receptor translocation to the plasma membrane. The Journal of Biological Chemistry. 2007;**282**:22278-22288

[11] Becerra-Díaz M, Strickland AB, Keselman A, Heller NM. Androgen and androgen receptor as enhancers of M2 macrophage polarization in allergic lung inflammation. Journal of Immunology. 2018;**201**(10):2923-2933. DOI: 10.4049/jimmunol.1800352

[12] Boorsma CE, Draijer C, Melgert BN. Macrophage heterogeneity in respiratory diseases. Mediators of Inflammation. 2013;**2013**:769214. DOI: 10.1155/2013/769214

[13] Nikonova A, Khaitov M, Jackson DJ, Traub S, Trujillo-Torralbo MB, Kudlay DA, et al. M1-like macrophages are potent producers of anti-viral interferons and M1-associated marker-positive lung macrophages are decreased during rhinovirus-induced asthma exacerbations. eBioMedicine.

2020;**54**:102734. DOI: 10.1016/j.ebiom.2020.102734

[14] Ford AQ, Dasgupta P, Mikhailenko I, Smith EM, Noben-Trauth N, Keegan AD. Adoptive transfer of IL-4Rα+ macrophages is sufficient to enhance eosinophilic inflammation in a mouse model of allergic lung inflammation. BMC Immunology. 2012;**13**:6. DOI: 10.1186/1471-2172-13-6

[15] Keselman A, Fang X, White PB, Heller NM. Estrogen signaling contributes to sex differences in macrophage polarization during asthma. Journal of Immunology. 2017;**199**(5):1573-1583. DOI: 10.4049/jimmunol.1601975

[16] Stone KC, Mercer RR, Gehr P, Stockstill B, Crapo JD. Allometric relationships of cell numbers and size in the mammalian lung. American Journal of Respiratory Cell and Molecular Biology. 1992;**6**:235-243

[17] Kousteni S, Bellido T, Plotkin LI, O'Brien CA, Bodenner DL, Han L, et al. Nongenotropic, sex-nonspecific signaling through the estrogen or androgen receptors: Dissociation from transcriptional activity. Cell. 2001;**104**:719-730

[18] Ojeda MS, Gómez NN, Gil E, Scardapane L, Gimenez MS. Morphologic and biochemical changes in castrated rat lung after surgical and pharmacological castration. Brazilian Journal of Medical and Biological Research. 2000;**33**:279-285

[19] Phaniendra A, Jestadi DB, Periyasamy L. Free radicals: Properties, sources, targets, and their implication in various diseases. Indian Journal of Clinical Biochemistry. 2015;**30**(1):11-26. DOI: 10.1007/s12291-014-0446-0

[20] Alvarez SM, Biaggio VS, Ciminari ME, Piguillem SN, Pacheco Guiñazú AB, Escobar Correas SM, et al. Androgen deprivation and cytoprotective parameters in rat lung. International Journal of Research Studies in Biosciences (IJRSB). 2015;**3**:150-163

[21] Bhattacharyya A, Chattopadhyay R, Mitra S, Crowe SE. Oxidative stress: An essential factor in the pathogenesis of gastrointestinal mucosal diseases. Physiological Reviews. 2014;**94**:329-354. DOI: 10.1152/physrev.00040.2012

[22] Rahal A, Kumar A, Singh V, Yadav B, Tiwari R, Chakraborty S, et al. Oxidative stress, prooxidants, and antioxidants: The interplay. BioMed Research International. 2014;**2014**:761264. DOI: 10.1155/2014/761264

[23] Di Meo S, Reed TT, Venditti P, Victor VM. Role of ROS and RNS sources in physiological and pathological conditions. Oxidative Medicine and Cellular Longevity. 2016;**2016**:1245049. DOI: 10.1155/2016/1245049

[24] Bassey IE, Emodi BA, Akpan UO, Iyakndue IFA, Anakebe EA, Icha BE, et al. Impact of androgen deprivation on oxidative stress and antioxidant status in Nigerian patients with prostate cancer undergoing androgen deprivation therapy. JCO Global Oncology. 2020;**6**:1481-1489. DOI: 10.1200/GO.20.00290

[25] Bassey IE, Ikpi DE, Isong IKP, Akpan UO, Onyeukwu CC, Nwankwo NP, et al. Effect of combined calcium, magnesium, vitamin C and E supplementation on seminal parameters and serum oxidative stress markers in fructose-induced diabetic Wistar rats. Archives of Physiology and Biochemistry. 2020;**25**:1-8. DOI: 10.1080/13813455.2020.1716017

[26] Ye Z, Liu W, Zhuo Q, Hu Q, Liu M, Sun Q, et al. Ferroptosis: Final destination for cancer? Cell Proliferation. 2020;**53**(3):e12761

[27] Nita M, Grzybowski A. The role of the reactive oxygen species and oxidative stress in the pathomechanism of the age-related ocular diseases and other pathologies of the anterior and posterior eye segments in adults. Oxidative Medicine and Cellular Longevity. 2016;**2016**:3164734. DOI: 10.1155/2016/3164734

[28] Cabello N, Mishra V, Sinha U, DiAngelo SL, Chroneos ZC, Ekpa NA, et al. Sex differences in the expression of lung inflammatory mediators in response to ozone. American Journal of Physiology. Lung Cellular and Molecular Physiology. 2015;**309**:L1150-L1163. DOI: 10.1152/ajplung.00018.2015

[29] Hu C, Yang J, Qi Z, Wu H, Wang B, Zou F, et al. Heat shock proteins: Biological functions, pathological roles, and therapeutic opportunities. MedComm (2020). 2022;**3**(3):e161. DOI: 10.1002/mco2.161

[30] Voltz JW, Card JW, Carey MA, Degraff LM, Ferguson CD, Flake GP, et al. Male sex hormones exacerbate lung function impairment after bleomycin-induced pulmonary fibrosis. American Journal of Respiratory Cell and Molecular Biology. 2008;**39**(1):45-52. DOI: 10.1165/rcmb.2007-0340OC

[31] Prakash YS. Emerging concepts in smooth muscle contributions to airway structure and function: Implications for health and disease. American Journal of Physiology. Lung Cellular and Molecular Physiology. 2016;**311**:L1113-L1140. DOI: 10.1152/ajplung.00370.2016

[32] Keselman A, Heller N. Estrogen signalling modulates allergic inflammation and contributes to sex differences in asthma. Frontiers in Immunology. 2015;**6**:568. DOI: 10.3389/fimmu.2015.00568

[33] Leffler J, Stumbles PA, Strickland DH. Immunological processes driving IgE sensitisation and disease development in males and females. International Journal of Molecular Sciences. 2018;**19**(6):E1554. DOI: 10.3390/ijms19061554

[34] Tamaki K, Sakihara E, Miyata H, Hirahara N, Kirichek O, Tawara R, et al. Utility of self-administered questionnaires for identifying individuals at risk of COPD in Japan: The OCEAN (Okinawa COPD case finding Assessment) study. International Journal of Chronic Obstructive Pulmonary Disease. 2021;**16**:1771-1782. DOI: 10.2147/COPD.S302259

[35] Ciminari ME, Pérez Chaca MV, Álvarez SM, Biaggio VS, Gómez NN. Analysis of the relationship between zinc deficiency, androgen disorders, and lung. In: Preedy V, Patel V, editors. Handbook of Famine, Starvation, and Nutrient Deprivation. Cham: Springer. pp 1931-1950. DOI: 10.1007/978-3-319-55387-0_90

[36] Paschos A, Pandya R, Duivenvoorden WC, Pinthus JH. Oxidative stress in prostate cancer: Changing research concepts towards a novel paradigm for prevention and therapeutics. Prostate Cancer and Prostatic Diseases. 2013;**16**:217-225. DOI: 10.1038/pcan.2013.13

[37] Rabe KF, Watz H, Baraldo S, Pedersen F, Biondini D, Bagul N, et al. Anti-inflammatory effects of roflumilast in chronic obstructive pulmonary disease (ROBERT): A 16-week, randomised, placebo-controlled trial. Lancet. 2018, 2018;**389**:1931-1940. DOI: 10.1016/S2213-2600(18)30331-X

[38] Kotlyarov S. Involvement of the Innate Immune System in the Pathogenesis of Chronic Obstructive Pulmonary Disease. International Journal of Molecular Sciences. 2022;**23**(2):985. DOI: 10.3390/ijms23020985

[39] Retamales I, Elliott WM, Meshi B, Coxson HO, Pare PD, Sciurba FC, et al. Amplification of inflammation in emphysema and its association with latent adenoviral infection. American Journal of Respiratory and Critical Care Medicine. 2001;**164**(3):469-473. DOI: 10.1164/ajrccm.164.3.2007149

[40] Wang X, Huang L, Jiang S, Cheng K, Wang D, Luo Q, et al. Testosterone attenuates pulmonary epithelial inflammation in male rats of COPD model through preventing NRF1-derived NF-kB signaling. Journal of Molecular Cell Biology. 2021;**13**(2):128-140. DOI: 10.1093/jmcb/mjaa079

[41] Bobjer J, Katrinaki M, Tsatsanis C, Lundberg Giwercman Y, Giwercman A. Negative association between testosterone concentration and inflammatory markers in young men: A nested cross-sectional study. PLoS One. 2013 Apr 18;**8**(4):e61466. DOI: 10.1371/journal.pone.0061466

[42] Tremellen K, McPhee N, Pearce K, Benson S, Schedlowski M, Engler H. Endotoxin-initiated inflammation reduces testosterone production in men of reproductive age. American Journal of Physiology. Endocrinology and Metabolism. 2018 Mar 1;**314**(3):E206-E213. DOI: 10.1152/ajpendo.00279.2017

[43] Hunt CD, Johnson PE, Herbel J, Mullen LK. Effects of dietary zinc depletion on seminal volume and zinc loss, serum testosterone concentrations, and sperm morphology in young men. The American Journal of Clinical Nutrition. 1992;**56**:148-157

[44] Hamdi SA, Nassif OI, Ardawi MS. Effect of marginal or severe dietary zinc deficiency on testicular development and functions of the rat. Archives of Andrology. 1997;**38**(3):243-253. DOI: 10.3109/01485019708994883

[45] Omu AE, Al-Azemi MK, Al-Maghrebi M, Mathew CT, Omu FE, Kehinde EO, et al. Molecular basis for the effects of zinc deficiency on spermatogenesis: An experimental study in the Sprague-Dawley rat model. Indian Journal of Urology. 2015;**31**(1):57-64. DOI: 10.4103/0970-1591.139570

[46] Hesketh JE. Effects of dietary zinc deficiency on Leydig cell ultrastructure in the boar. Journal of Comparative Pathology. 1982;**92**:239-247

[47] Kambe T, Hashimoto A, Fujimoto S. Current understanding of ZIP and ZnT zinc transporters in human health and diseases. Cellular and Molecular Life Sciences. 2014;**71**:3281-3295

[48] Chu Q, Chi Z-H, Zhang X, Liang D, Wang X, Zhao Y, Zhang L, Zhang P. A potential role for zinc transporter 7 in testosterone synthesis in mouse Leydig tumor cells. International Journal of Molecular Medicine 2016, 37(6): 1619-1626. https://doi.org/10.3892/ijmm.2016.2576

[49] Shaffer PL, Jivan A, Dollins DE, Claessens F, Gewirth DT. Structural basis of androgen receptor binding to selective androgen response elements. Proceedings of the National Academy of Sciences of the United States of America. 2004;**101**:4758-4763

[50] Biaggio VS, Alvarez-Olmedo D, Perez Chaca MV, Salvetti NR, Valdez SR, Fanelli MA, et al. Cytoprotective mechanisms in rats lung parenchyma with zinc deprivation. Biometals. 2014;**27**:305-315

[51] Scully EP, Haverfield J, Ursin RL, Tannenbaum C, Klein SL. Considering how biological sex impacts immune responses and COVID-19 outcomes. Nature Reviews. Immunology. 2020;**20**:442-447

[52] Cutolo M, Smith V, Paolino S. Understanding immune effects of estrogens to explain the reduced morbidity and mortality in female versus male COVID-19 patients. Comparisons with autoimmunity and vaccination. Clinical and Experimental Rheumatology. 2020;**38**:383-386

[53] Nie X, Qian L, Sun R, et al. Multi-organ proteomic landscape of COVID-19 autopsies. Cell. 2021;**184**:775-791

[54] Sher T, Dy GK, Adjei AA. Small cell lung cancer. Mayo Clinic Proceedings. 2008;**83**:355-367

[55] Noguchi M, Morikawa A, Kawasaki M, et al. Small adenocarcinoma of the lung. Histologic characteristics and prognosis. Cancer. 1995;**75**:2844-2852

[56] Zappa C, Mousa SA. Non-small cell lung cancer: Current treatment and future advances. Translational Lung Cancer Research. 2016;**5**(3):288-300 DOI: 10.21037/tlcr.2016.06.07

[57] Muscat JE, Stellman SD, Zhang ZF, et al. Cigarette smoking and large cell carcinoma of the lung. Cancer Epidemiology, Biomarkers & Prevention. 1997;**6**:477-480

[58] Chan YX, Alfonso H, Chubb SA, Handelsman DJ, Fegan PG, Hankey GJ, et al. Higher dihydrotestosterone is associated with the incidence of lung cancer in older men. Hormones and Cancer. 2017 Apr;**8**(2):119-126. DOI: 10.1007/s12672-017-0287-4

[59] Harlos C, Musto G, Lambert P, Ahmed R, Pitz MW. Androgen pathway manipulation and survival in patients with lung cancer. Horm Cancer. 2015 Jun;**6**(2-3):120-127. DOI: 10.1007/s12672-015-0218-1 Epub 2015 Mar 20

[60] Pantazopoulos I, Magounaki K, Kotsiou O, Rouka E, Perlikos F, Kakavas S, et al. Incorporating biomarkers in COPD management: The research keeps going. Journal of Personalized Medicine. 2022 Mar 1;**12**(3):379. DOI: 10.3390/jpm12030379

[61] Antus B. Oxidative stress markers in sputum. Oxidative Medicine and Cellular Longevity. 2016;**2016**:2930434. DOI: 10.1155/2016/2930434

Chapter 6

Benefits of Testosterone Replacement and Methods of Substitution

Kenneth W.K. Ho

Abstract

Testosterone substitution and replacement therapy is effective for managing testosterone deficiency. Traditional routes of administration include oral, nasal, transdermal, and intramuscular. Scrotal application of testosterone cream has been made recently available. Physician's choice of one preparation over another is based on testosterone bioavailability, side effect profile and ability to achieve therapeutic levels. Patient's choice is influenced by comfort, ease of use and product acceptability. This is important for compliance and achievement of good outcomes. Testosterone substitution can be overused and associated with adverse effects. Individuals at risk are older, obese with chronic cardiorespiratory disorders, and lower urinary tract symptoms. Therapeutic monitoring is vital and is achieved through measuring serum total testosterone levels and clinical follow-up. Decision on therapy outcomes should be individualised, based on symptom control and testosterone effects on organ function. Supra-therapeutic testosterone levels should be avoided as adverse outcomes such as worsening obstructive sleep apnoea, polycythaemia, and prostatic growth stimulation are more likely.

Keywords: routes of administration, monitoring of efficacy, adverse effects, individualised therapy, non-testosterone options

1. Introduction

In males, testosterone production occurs under the control of the hypothalamic-pituitary-testicular (HPT) axis. The gonadotropin pulse generator awakens in the lead up to puberty, driving the development of the testes, with the follicular stimulating hormone (FSH) responsible for the development of the seminiferous tubules and the luteinising hormone (LH), the production of testosterone from testicular Leydig cells. The release of gonadotropins results in enlargement of the testes, and a pair of 4 ml testes signals the start of puberty. The surge in testosterone that follows puberty is responsible for the eventual male phenotype characterised by voice deepening, body hair development, muscular and skeletal growth. Other secondary sexual characteristics include lengthening of the penis, pubic and scrotal hair. Testosterone primes the skeletal response to growth hormone (GH) stimulation and results in the growth spurt that follows puberty. Spermatogenesis arises from FSH stimulating spermatogonia development and spermatozoa production. Testosterone production is regulated via the hypothalamus-pituitary-testicular axis. Regulation of gonadotropin secretion from the gonadotroph cells in the anterior pituitary occurs through stimulation by gonadotropin-releasing hormone (GnRH) from the hypothalamus. The gonadotroph cells have testosterone (T) and estrogen (E2) receptors that receive negative inhibition from testosterone and oestradiol respectively [1].

Understanding this feedback response pathway allows the clinician to determine the cause of testicular failure. In primary testicular failure, testicular hypofunction results in the fall of testosterone levels and the consequent reduction of feedback inhibition of the hypothalamus and pituitary, result in a corresponding rise of LH and FSH. The causes of testicular hypofunction include destruction of testes through mumps, testicular cancer, alkylating chemotherapeutic agents, and orchidectomies. In secondary testicular failure, disruption of the HPT axis occurs at the hypothalamus and/or pituitary level. Some examples are large sellar tumours that compress on the pituitary, causing irreparable damage to the gonadotroph cells or damage to the pituitary after debulking of large sellar tumours. In such situations, the reduction of LH leads to very low testosterone levels. It is uncommon for direct hypothalamic injury to cause secondary testicular failure. More commonly, secondary testicular failure occurs when supraphysiological doses of testosterone are administered for prolonged periods, resulting in suppression of gonadotropins. When the supraphysiological testosterone doses are stopped, LH and FSH levels remain very low and may take months to recover.

Testosterone has an anabolic effect on cell growth and is important for skeletal and muscular development. Once biosynthesised and released by the testes, testosterone is transported in the blood, bound to sex hormone binding globulin (SHBG) with a small unbound portion (2%), as free testosterone. Around 95% of circulating testosterone reaches the target cells and exerts its effects by entering the cytoplasm and binding to the androgen receptors (ARs). The AR is widely distributed among reproductive and nonreproductive tissues, including the prostate, and seminal vesicles, external genitalia, skin, testes, cartilage, sebaceous glands, hair follicles, sweat glands, cardiac muscle, skeletal muscle and smooth muscle, gastrointestinal vesicular cells, thyroid follicular cells, adrenal cortex, liver, pineal and many cortical and subcortical regions, including spinal motor neurons [2]. The testosterone-AR complex results in rapid cellular signalling cascades via SRC/MAPK/ERK pathways that lead to cell proliferation and survival or enter the nucleus and bind to AR elements on target genes to increase gene expression. About 10% of testosterone is converted to dihydrotestosterone (DHT) via 5 α-reductase activity in the genitals, prostate, and skin. DHT is several times more potent than testosterone and is vital for the sexual differentiation of male genitalia during embryonic development [3]. Approximately 0.1% of testosterone is converted into estrogens by aromatase (CYP19A1) activity in bone, fat, or brain, where testosterone exerts its anabolic activity via the estrogen receptor (ER). All these hormones (testosterone, DHT and estrogens) exert negative feedback on the HPT axis [4].

In men, testosterone levels can vary widely, from very low levels late at night to peak levels in late morning. This is because the pituitary releases LH in a pulsatile manner, dependent upon periods of light and sleep. Normal ranges in healthy eugonadal men vary widely. This may be dependent on ethnic, genetic, and geographical factors. It is also affected by acute and chronic ill health. Total testosterone was determined in a reference sample of 456 healthy young men, (19–40 years), using Liquid Chromatography Tandem Mass Spectrometry, demonstrating that the 2.5 percentile cut-off was 12.1 nmol/l (348.3 ng/dl) and the 97.5 percentile was 41.5 nmol/l

(1196.6 ng/dl). In very healthy men aged 70-89 years, the reference interval using mass spectrometry was 6.4–25.7 nmol/l (184.6-741.2 ng/dL) [5]. Men who describe hypogonadal symptoms but have testosterone levels at the lower limit of the normal eugonadal range, are thought to have functional hypogonadism. They may also have chronic disease or are obese. Clinical testosterone deficiency syndrome, or hypogonadism, refers to a spectrum of symptoms that include physical, psychological, and sexual. Hypogonadal men may report significant fatigue, and muscle weakness, as well as feelings of reduced motivation, and low mood. More commonly, sexual symptoms predominate, such as reduced libido, or disinterest in sexual relations, and poor erections. Hypogonadism is often associated with obesity in a bi-directional causal relationship. Chronically low testosterone levels may predispose to muscle atrophy and fat gain, whilst obesity is thought to exert an inhibitory effect on the gonadotrophs in the anterior pituitary and on the GnRH cells in the hypothalamus. The associations of fatigue with chronically low testosterone are multifactorial and include psychological aspects such as depression and low motivation, but also that of chronic normocytic anaemia, due to reduced erythropoiesis.

When there is clear evidence of primary or secondary testicular dysfunction, i.e., hypogonadal symptoms, associated with persistently low testosterone levels, testosterone replacement or substitution is wholly justified, as hypogonadal symptoms should respond well to intervention. However, where hypogonadal symptoms occur outside these situations, there are differences of opinion as to when testosterone therapy is initiated. An international survey of adult endocrinologists in 2015 indicated that in men with hypogonadal symptoms, 42.4% of endocrinologists surveyed would treat with testosterone replacement [6]. A placebo controlled double blinded randomised controlled trial (RCT) in >65-year-old hypogonadal men with total testosterone level below 9.5 nmol/l (275 ng/dl) showed that raising the total testosterone level to that of mid-normal range for 19–40-year-old men, significantly improved sexual function, and mood, but not vitality or walking distance [7]. Therefore, hypogonadal men with testosterone levels below 9.5 nmol/l (275 ng/dl) may be considered acceptable for testosterone therapy in the absence of correctable lifestyle factors.

2. Effects of testosterone substitution or replacement therapy

Previous observational studies have suggested that testosterone replacement therapy (TRT) may lead to increased cardiovascular risks, but recent prospective studies have not found this to be so. In contrast these studies have suggested that TRT may be beneficial in reducing the metabolic derangements associated with type 2 diabetes. In a prospective treatment study, 178 such patients with normal baseline testosterone of 12 nmol/l (346.1 ng/dl), were given testosterone undecanoate (TU) and compared with similar patients who did not choose to receive TRT. The TRT group had shown reductions in HbA1c, fasted insulin, fasted glucose levels compared to the matched group who did not receive therapy [8]. Such findings were supported in the recently published T4DM study, which had randomised obese men with the metabolic syndrome to TU depot injection compared to placebo over 6 months and found significant reductions in fasted glucose, reduced abdominal fat mass, and increased muscle mass [9].

Hypogonadal men report reduction in libido and erections, energy, strength and endurance, enjoyment of life, mood, mental concentration, and work performance. TRT is associated with improvement in these areas. The Androgen Deficiency in Ageing Males

(ADAM) [10] is a research tool developed by the St. Louis University to assess hypogonadism. The International Index of Erectile Function (IIEF-5) evaluate erectile dysfunction (ED) through measures in erectile function, orgasmic function, sexual desire, intercourse satisfaction and overall sexual function [11]. Studies have shown reduction of ADAM scores and improvement in IIEF-5 scores in hypogonadal men who receive TRT.

Hypogonadal men experience significant changes to their body composition. Administration of androgen deprivation therapy for prostate cancer leads to sustained muscle loss and fat gain, most profound in the first 12 months [12]. The effects can be reversed with testosterone replacement [13], with dual energy X-ray absorptiometry (DEXA) showing reduction in fat mass and increased muscle mass. Loss of lean muscle mass is associated with ageing in men. TRT in men with sarcopenia has been associated with increase in lean muscle mass but the effects on strength and overall quality of life have been inconsistent [14]. Hypogonadal men have a significant risk of secondary osteoporosis [15]. It has been shown that in men who received androgen deprivation therapy, there is increased bone turnover and 2.5% decrease in bone mineral density annually [16]. In a subsequent sub-study of the T4DM, the T4Bone study had shown that TRT may be associated with significantly increased volumetric bone mineral density in cortical bone in obese metabolic men.

Testosterone activates the amygdala enhancing its emotional activity and its resistance to pre-frontal restraining control [17]. Aggressive behaviour arises through interaction between the amygdala and the hypothalamus which brings about emotions which the prefontal cognitive centres then modulate and control. Testosterone is important for psychological maturation of the brain during puberty, which results in anatomical and organisational changes in the male brain. Hypogonadal men often report lack of motivation and often feel low in mood. These symptoms may be due to the physical effects of low testosterone on muscle and bone function. Testosterone replacement can exert profound psychological effects. Testosterone replacement for 51 hypogonadal men (age 22–60 years) with baseline level <8.3 nmol/l (250 ng/dl) over 60 days led to significantly decreases in anger, sadness, irritability, tiredness, nervousness, and improvement in energy, friendliness, and sense of well-being [18]. The levels of testosterone and DHT correlated with improvement on initial treatment, but once therapeutic level was achieved, further escalation of testosterone no longer correlated with improvement.

3. Methods of testosterone substitution

In ancient times, ingested animal testicular extracts were known to bestow improved vitality and to act as an aphrodisiac [19]. In the early 1900s, injected testicular transplants from goats, ram, deer, boar and bulls were used and even testicles of executed criminals were used to substitute for males with sexual dysfunction [19]. From 1935, synthesis of testosterone from cholesterol became possible and led to the award of the Nobel Prize for Chemistry in 1939 [19]. Testosterone was first trialled as oral administration, but because of extensive first pass metabolism by the liver, it became necessary to alkylate the 17-hydroxy position, giving rise to androgens that are more resistant to hepatic metabolism. 17α-methyl-testosterone was introduced in 1939 by Foss and became extensively used for its androgenic and protein anabolic effects. It can be ingested orally or administered via trans buccal route [20]. After several decades of use however, it was found to cause cholestatic jaundice, reversible hepatotoxicity, and some cases of death, ending its use in the 1980s [21].

3.1 Intramuscular injections

With the problems encountered from first pass metabolism and hepatotoxicity, other alterations were made to the testosterone molecule to make testosterone administration more effective and safer. Adding an ester moiety to the 17-hydroxy position of synthetic testosterone made it hydrophobic, so it may be stored in oil and injected intramuscularly [22]. Intramuscular injections have been used from early and are currently still one of the most popular modes of administering testosterone. It results in an effective rise in testosterone levels with suppression of gonadotropins, resulting in symptomatic response. Examples are testosterone propionate, testosterone cypionate, testosterone enanthate, and TU. There are significant differences in elimination half-lives, with testosterone propionate being the shortest at 0.8 days, testosterone enanthate 4.5 days, and TU 33.9 days [23]. Testosterone propionate was first used in 1939. Administration of a single dose of 50 mg testosterone propionate led to a supraphysiological peak of 40.2 nmol/l (1159.4 ng/dL) 14 hours later, but quickly returned to below baseline on day 3 (57 hours) after injection, with the troughs between 3-7 nmol/L (86.5-201.9 ng/dL) [24]. Therefore, based on the pharmacokinetics of a single dose, testosterone propionate will have to be injected intramuscularly every 3rd day i.e. twice a week, which would not be practical for long term substitution. In addition, it is associated with peaks as high as 45 nmol/l (1297.9 ng/dL) and troughs of 3 nmol/l (86.5 ng/dL) [23]. It is now administered in a mixture of esters (propionate, phenylpropionate, isocaproate, and decanoate) marketed as Sustanon. However, it became superseded by the longer-acting testosterone enanthate.

Testosterone enanthate was first manufactured in the mid 1950s [25], and is still commonly used, popular among body builders. Snyder et al [26]. tested the efficacy of testosterone enanthate for treating male primary hypogonadism and determined that the regimens most practical in terms of injection interval and yet effective in suppressing LH to normal levels, were 200 mg every 2 weeks or 300 mg every 3 weeks. Salmimies et al administered fortnightly injections of testosterone enanthate in a range of doses from 50 to 250 mg, to hypogonadal males with a variety of aetiologies such as testicular, pituitary, or hypothalamic failure. They documented their sexual behaviour via questionnaires. In general, improvements in sexual desire, erectile frequencies and ejaculations were dose dependent. However, the treatment threshold below which hypogonadal symptoms were to occur was wide, from 6.9 nmol/l (200 ng/dL) to 15.6 nmol/l (450 ng/dL) [27]. Testosterone cypionate has a similar pharmacokinetic profile to testosterone enanthate. Intramuscular injection of 200 mg testosterone cypionate leads to a peak of 38.5 $\pm$ 15.3 nmol/l (1108 $\pm$ 440 ng/dl) from 2 to 3 days and progressively decline from day 5 to pre-injection baseline at 14 days [28]. There is a corresponding peak and decline in free testosterone and oestradiol levels. The frequency of injections every 2–3 weeks for both testosterone esters and the wide testosterone fluctuations makes it less than ideal for long term use.

TU was synthesised in the 1970s by adding the undecyclic acid to the C17β position of testosterone. When administered orally, it is absorbed via gut lymphatics and therefore by-passes the liver. After reaching the blood circulation, it undergoes de-esterification, releasing the unmodified testosterone [29]. It was first used orally and provided a safe non-injected method of administering testosterone that bypassed the liver and circumvented the issues of liver toxicity [30]. In 1980s, the World Health Organisation sponsored a Special Programme of Research, Development and Research Training in Human Reproduction which developed an injectable TU prepared in tea seed oil and introduced in the late 1990s. When administered as a

500 or 1000 mg dose, it resulted in a peak of 47.8 ± 10.1 nmol/l (1379 ± 291 ng/dL) and 54.2 ± 4.8 nmol/l (1563 ± 138 ng/dL) at the end of 7 days and declined to baseline by 6–8 weeks, showing an elimination half-life of 18.3 ± 2.3 days and 23.7 ± 2.7 days respectively [31]. It was first trialled in China with repeated 500 mg in 4 ml injections every 6–8 weeks. A newer more concentrated formulation was later developed by Jenapharm/Schering, in which 1000 mg of TU was completely dissolved in benzyl benzoate, diluted in 4 ml of refined castor oil and delivered in a vial [32].

In the initial pharmacokinetics studies carried out at Munster, Germany, a single injection of 1000 mg of TU resulted in peak testosterone level of 22.2 ± 2.0 nmol/l (640 ± 57.7 ng/dL) at 7–14 days, with levels >10 nmol/l (288 ng/dL) for up to 8 weeks. When 1000 mg was given every 6 weeks for 5 months, there was steady accumulation of testosterone to 40.8 ± 3.8 mmol/l (1177 ± 109.6 ng/dL) at 6 months. There was a significant slow and steady rise of DHT and oestradiol levels and slight decline in SHBG levels. FSH and LH were suppressed at the end of the 6-month study. There was a significant slight increase in prostate volume, but it remained low [33]. Therefore, the optimal regimen of administrating TU is to give the first two injections 6 weeks apart and thereafter, the injection interval could be 10–14 weeks depending on the trough testosterone levels [32, 33]. It was first marketed at the end of 2003 in Europe, Latin America, and in Asia as Nebido (Bayer) and in Spain and Australia as Reandron 1000 (Bayer). It is available in a 4 ml vial with a concentration of 250 mg/ml formulation. Another TU injectable formulation Aveed (Endo Pharmaceuticals Solutions Inc.) was launched in the USA in 2010 as a single 3 ml ampoule containing 750 mg of TU. The 3 ml injection was given at baseline, 4 weeks later and then maintained at 10 weeks intervals. During a multicentre US based study the on-treatment troughs through a 64 week duration ranged from 10.8 to 13.5 nmol/l (309.6–389.8 ng/dl), and free testosterone, SHBG, DHT and oestradiol remained constant, while LH and FSH were suppressed [34].

3.2 Testosterone implants

Subdermal implant techniques were originally developed in the late 1930s and were first used to deliver testosterone pellets made up of compressed testosterone and cholesterol in the early 1950s. It has been in clinical use for >50 years, but its popularity waxed and waned during the 1980s into the 21st century. The technique and follow up procedures have been well described by Handelsman et al [35]. Implants are administered under sterile conditions by an experienced operator with an assistant, in a routine office setting using stainless steel wide-bore trocar (7.5 French gauge, 5 mm ID, 7 cm length), cannula and obturator set. Implants are placed subdermally in the lower abdominal wall lateral to or just about the level of the umbilicus. The supine patient's abdominal skin is prepped anti-septically and draped. Following a local anaesthetic injection, a small incision is made (0.5–1.0 cm) at least 5 cm from the midline, to allow introduction of the trocar. This permits the insertion of four 200 mg testosterone pellets radiating subdermally from the initial incision site, expelled from the trocar by the obturator at 5–10 cm from the puncture site. The puncture wound is closed without suture using adhesive sterile strips and covered by a clear, waterproof adhesive dressing, left in place for 5–7 days and removed by the patient. Subsequent implantations are usually scheduled every 4–6 months, but patients are generally reviewed in-between with or without testosterone levels. Most patients have no side effects and there is a high continuation rate of >90% over a decade. Main adverse events are minor infections, and oozing or minor bleeding, and extrusion of pellets as a result. The risk predictors for adverse events are increased physical activity at work, number of pellets inserted, and thinness of patients, who make the technique more difficult because of reduced subcutaneous fat.

Jockenhovel studied the pharmacokinetics of a single subdermal implantation of T-pellets in 14 hypogonadal men with baseline testosterone level below 3.6 nmol/l (103.8 ng/dL) [36]. Following implantation, there was a rapid rise of testosterone level to about 49 nmol/l (1413.3 ng/dL) within 2 days, followed by a plateau phase for a month, and a gradual decline to baseline by 12 months. Mean serum testosterone was below 10 nmol/l (288.4 ng/dL), after 6 months. Rise in serum DHT correlated with the initial rise of serum testosterone levels, but the DHT/testosterone ratio decreased after the implantation and was significantly below baseline from day 21 to 189. SHBG demonstrated a rapid decline in response to T-pellets but returned to baseline by day 300. Both LH and FSH were rapidly and markedly suppressed by testosterone pellet implantation, recovering towards their baseline by 6 months. Again, the adverse events are low, and relatively minor, and most men are happy to continue. A potential disadvantage is the rapid and extreme peak of testosterone after implantation and its implications on prostate growth. The other consideration is a degree of training and experience is needed for the procedure. However, the pellets are relatively inexpensive.

3.3 Oral administration

Current versions are available as TU administered in softgel capsules. There are several trade names, Andriol, Jatenza, and Tlando. Clinical studies have suggested oral preparations to be effective. Serum testosterone levels have increased by more than 50% after several months of daily use. This was associated with improvement in ADAM questionnaire scores and AMS scale, but not SF-36 scale [37]. Oral TU rely on absorption via gut lymphatics and should be administered twice or thrice with meal, preferably with some fat content. Gut absorption can therefore be subjective and contributes to testosterone level fluctuations. However, it is generally a safe option for use in older men, especially if prostate specific antigen (PSA) needs to be carefully followed.

Other oral preparations include administration of 30 mg testosterone via a sustained and controlled transbuccal route [38]. This involves the application of a small tablet pressed firmly onto the gums of the upper incisors for about 30 seconds, twice daily. The adhered tablet absorbs saliva to form a gel and is subsequently absorbed into the mucosa. It leads to a steady rise of testosterone levels to between 10 nmol/L (288.4 ng/dL) and 20 nmol/l (576.8 ng/dL). Upon cessation of therapy, baseline levels are returned after 14 days. Adherence to therapy is reasonably good, with >60% compliance. However, it is not a popular mode of replacement and is not widely available in many countries except in North America. Common issues are gum mucosa irritation.

3.4 Transdermal applications

There are several methods whereby testosterone can be administered topically. These can be done transdermally via scrotal (Testoderm), or non-scrotal skin patches (Androderm) or by transdermal hydroalcoholic gel (AndroGel or Testogel), or by creams (AndroForte). Transdermal patches were first used on the scrotal skin in 1987 [39]. It was a logical choice as the scrotal skin has the thinnest stratum corneum, which would allow easy penetration. However subsequent issues with poor adhesiveness, and the need for regular shaving and excessive DHT levels, made it an unpopular choice among clinicians and patients. Non-scrotal patches were trialled [40–42], and but required an effective alcohol-based excipient to allow adequate permeation of the testosterone through the thicker stratum corneum. This resulted in frequent skin irritation and often burn-like reactions [43]. It too fell out of favour.

In 2010, the FDA had approved a unique product containing 2% *w/v* testosterone dissolved in a solvent mixture of ethanol and isopropanol. The testosterone solution was provided in a bottle with a metered dose pump and a detachable applicator. A metered dose delivers 1.5 ml (equivalent to 30 mg of testosterone) into the applicator, which the patient then uses to rub the solution onto the axilla, and then allow the solution to evaporate after 3 minutes. The procedure is then repeated on the other axilla. The testosterone solution also contains octisalate which aids in the permeability of transdermal testosterone. This product was effective in restoring total testosterone levels to the normal range after 15 days in most individuals, with improvement in hypogonadal symptoms, through two metered doses (60 mg) daily [44]. The men were instructed to avoid having their partners or children touch their axillary areas as traces of testosterone can be recovered after application. However, for unspecified reasons, this product was removed from the market in 2017.

Testosterone transdermal gels were introduced in the early 2000s. Over the last 10 years, the product was marketed as a hydroalcoholic gel containing 1% (10 mg/g) of testosterone, delivered via metered actuations each containing 12.5 mg of testosterone. The standard daily dose was four to eight actuations (50–100 mg), with the starting dose at 50 mg, and increased as needed in consultation with their doctors, up to 100 mg daily. Bodily sites where the patients could apply the gel include the shoulders, upper arms, chest, and upper torso areas. The gel was applied in the morning, after a shower if needed, and the applied areas allowed to dry thoroughly (within minutes) and covered with clothing appropriately to prevent inadvertent transference to others. Testosterone levels were elevated into the eugonadal range with appropriate suppression of gonadotropins and was associated with improvements in mood, sexual function, satisfaction, and body composition. Adverse events were acceptably low, at 5.5%, and were mainly from mild skin erythema [43]. Testogel has been a highly marketed product and enjoys popularity world-wide.

Testosterone is also available as a 5% (50 mg/ml) alcohol-free topical testosterone cream (AndroForte 5). The T cream was supplied with a dose measuring applicator graduated in 0.5 ml increments. Patients can start with 2 ml (100 mg) with a maximum dose of 4 ml (200 mg) of cream massaged evenly over the skin of the torso daily. The dose can be adjusted over 3 months with consultation of their doctors. The treatment is effective in raising testosterone levels into the eugonadal range with appropriate lowering of gonadotropins. It is comparable to the use of Testogel with no difference in adverse events between the two products [45]. AndroForte 5 may also be administered as a scrotal skin application. Iyer et al. have shown effective elevation of testosterone levels with just a low dose of 12.5 mg (0.25 ml) and is comparable to that of 100 mg (2 ml) applied onto the abdominal skin [46]. This suggests that an eight-fold increase in bioavailability is attained via the scrotal skin route, which as discussed, has a thin stratum corneum and also has a high concentration of 5α reductase levels, which converts testosterone to DHT levels. Patients generally start with 0.5 ml (25 mg) massaged into the scrotum daily. There is no need to remove scrotal hair as the cream is well absorbed into the scrotum. The daily dose can be increased by 0.25 ml up to 0.75 ml if needed over 3–6 months in consultation with medical practitioners. This therefore provides an economical yet effective way of testosterone substitution.

3.5 Nasal delivery

Another method of delivery that has been generally available in North America since 2015 is that of nasal testosterone gel. Natesto is a 4.5% testosterone thixotropic gel applied intranasally by delivering 5.5 mg via a metered dose pump, into each nostril two or three times a day. In an open-label dose titration study, that included overweight men (mean age 54 years) with late-onset (functional) hypogonadism, 306 were randomly assigned to either twice or thrice daily regimens [47]. Patient responses were quantified using the IIEF and the Positive and Negative Effect Schedule (PANAS) at baseline and at 30-day intervals for 3 months. Regardless of the baseline total testosterone levels, which can range from <3.4 nmol/l (<100 ng/dl) to 27.3 nmol/l (800 ng/dl), administration of Natesto led to a rapid rise of total testosterone to about 24.4–27.3 nmol/l (700–800 ng/dl) after an hour but returns to baseline after 6 hours. At day 90 of treatment, there were corresponding rises in IIEF scores of about 40%, irrespective of the baseline pre-treatment total testosterone levels and an increase in positive PANAS and decrease in negative PANAS scores. In a dose titration study, patients were started with a divided daily dose of 22 mg but may be titrated to 33 mg depending on symptoms at day 90. The majority stayed on 22 mg daily, whilst a third of patients preferred the 33 mg daily dose [48]. Symptoms were recorded using the qADAM, and patient satisfaction was documented at baseline, and at 30 day intervals up to 120 days. It has been generally well accepted with most citing convenience and ease of use, effectiveness, travel friendliness, but also listing nasal drip as a potential deterrent to using it [48].

4. Testosterone substitution in sports

Testosterone's potent anabolic effects on musculoskeletal and bone marrow quickly led to widespread illicit use in sports [49, 50]. Testosterone propionate's half-life of 2–3 weeks makes it popular as an ideal anabolic steroid to enhance athletic performance. It became implicated in illicit steroid use and doping scandals in sport use [51]. The advent of mandatory and sophisticated drug testing at international competitions have not eliminated the illicit use of testosterone rather, anabolic steroid use have found themselves into other lesser competitive sporting events such as in high schools and clubs [52]. Individuals have reportedly used testosterone and other anabolic steroids in a pre-specified period leading up to the competition. Giorgi et al have shown that testosterone enanthate administered at supraphysiologic doses at 3.5 mg/kg/week over 12 weeks (approximately 300 mg/week) was associated with improved physical conditioning, doubling of muscle strength and increased weight over placebo. However, upon withdrawal of testosterone injections, the enhancements did not continue, and subjects would return to their baseline 12 weeks after cessation, despite ongoing training [53]. Concerningly, youths are turning to anabolic steroids to enhance not only their physical performance but also their physical appearance [54].

5. Opioid induced androgen deficiency

Individuals who use opioids for long term are at risk of developing hypogonadism [55]. Activation of μ-receptors in the hypothalamic pituitary axis can result in suppression of the gonadal axis. The prevalence of opioid induced androgen deficiency varies from 19% to 86% depending on the testosterone threshold for defining hypogonadism. The true incidence is likely to be higher than reported as the association is under-recognised by clinicians. The risk is higher in chronic opioid users, with a Morphine Equivalent Dose of greater than 60 mg, but shorter use duration with the more potent and long-acting opioids such as fentanyl are at higher risk. On the hand, opioids with partial μ-receptor agonism such as buprenorphine or tapentadol have lower risks. Affected individuals report sexual dysfunction, depression, reduced fertility, reduced bone health, increased weight, and elevated cardiovascular risks. Testosterone replacement can be achieved via topical or parenteral routes, with benefits in reduction of pain perception, and opioid dosing, improvement in libido, body composition, and bone density.

6. Testosterone for male transgender (transmen) management

Testosterone is the key hormone for adult individuals with Gender Dysphoria, who want to transition from being a female to male. Transmen who receive testosterone substitution develop amenorrhoea, increased muscle mass and strength, male pattern body hair and deepening of voice. The US Endocrine Society recommends maintaining serum testosterone within the normal male range of 11.1–34.7 nmol/l (320–1000 ng/dl) [56]. Testosterone substitution methods have included oral, transdermal, and parenteral routes. Pelusi et al [57]. studied testosterone substitution in 45 transmen over a year and randomised them to combined T. propionate/enanthate esters intramuscular injections every 10 days, or daily testosterone gel application or T. undecanoate depot 12 weekly deep intramuscular injections. All three groups report amenorrhoea by the first year of treatment and increased lean mass and reduced fat mass. There were significant changes in lipid profiles without cardiovascular outcomes. All study subjects reported general life satisfaction at 1 year but over time, all of study subjects moved over to maintenance TU treatment. A retrospective 5-year review of 50 transmen between 21 and 42 years of age comparing T undecanoate 1000 mg IMI every 12 weeks with T enanthate 250 mg IMI every 3–4 weeks showed similar results in metabolic and anthropometric parameters. Serum testosterone rose from 1.4 ± 0.6 (40.4 ± 17.3 ng/dL) to 1.9 ± 0.8 nmol/l (54.8 ± 23.1 ng/dL) at baseline to range between 12.1 ± 3.8 nmol/L (350.0 ± 109.6 ng/dL) and 20.8 ± 11.4 nmol/l (599.9 ± 328.8 ng/dL) over the 5 years. There were consistent reports of improved life satisfaction through attainment of their desired male phenotype. Though there were significantly deranged lipid profiles, there are no reports of increased cardiovascular mortality in transmen within two decades of therapy [58].

7. Testosterone substitution pitfalls and monitoring requirements

With improved testosterone assays, the challenge of testosterone therapy is to find substitution routes that not only ensure a consistent testosterone delivery but also allow safe therapeutic monitoring and prevent transference to others. Currently the options are oral administration via the oro-gastric route, trans-buccal, transdermal gels, transdermal patches, deep intramuscular injections, and subcutaneous dermal implants. WHO recommendations for the ideal TRT preparation are that it must be safe, effective in correcting symptoms and consequences of T deficiency, inexpensive, of easy administration, with good release profile, ensuring reproducible circulating levels of T and prolonged duration of action, flexible dosing and able to maintain normal physiologic levels of testosterone. Side effects relate to the excessive peaks and troughs. They include acne, injection pain, and nerve injury. Other unintended consequences are potentially reducing male fertility, worsening sleep apnoea, increased haematocrit and precipitation of polycythaemia, prostatic hyperplasia, un-masking of undiagnosed prostatic cancer and breast cancer, the rare pulmonary oil microembolism (POME), and anaphylaxis.

Careful attention should be given to older men, those with prostate hypertrophy, obese men who are at risk of sleep apnoea, or unstable coronary artery disease. Testosterone therapy may unmask sleep apnoea, and if untreated, may precipitate polycythaemia. It is recommended to keep haematocrit <54%. Prostatic hyperplasia during testosterone therapy is usually not a problem if done carefully. It is prudent to start with short-acting preparations such as testosterone gels or short-acting testosterone enanthate in men with moderate risk. Consider digital rectal examination in at-risk men, for example those with family history of prostate cancer, between 55 and 69 years of age. PSA must be measured at baseline, prior to starting and 6 monthly during TRT. However, after initial 12 months of documented safety, PSA may be monitored once every 12 months. Younger or pre-pubertal males are particularly sensitive to the psychological and sexualising effects of testosterone, so it is prudent to start with low doses and to increase slowly [59]. Testosterone therapy is also contraindicated in males with hepatocyte tumours because of its stimulatory effects on Cyclin E kinase activity potentially driving carcinogenesis [60].

Patients should be counselled on the risks versus benefits of testosterone therapy. Testosterone therapy can be done effectively and safely. The various options are discussed with the patient, and the most suitable route of administration decided, based on the effectiveness, safety of monitoring, drug access, cost, and patient acceptability. Patients should be reviewed at 3–6 monthly intervals. Assessment of efficacy and side effects along with therapeutic monitoring should be done at each visit. This involves assessing testosterone levels, LH, FSH, and PSA levels. Testosterone levels often correlate with symptom improvement, but maintenance of low normal trough testosterone levels maybe important for prevention of over treatment and drug toxicity. It is particularly pertinent in long acting (depot) preparations such as intramuscular TU.

8. Non-testosterone substitution options

8.1 Tribulus terrestris

Non-testosterone herbal extracts may have a role in treating ED and male hypoactive sexual desire disorder (HSDD). Tribulus terrestris or commonly known as Puncture Vine, have been used for thousands of years in Asiatic cultures as an aphrodisiac. The plant contains steroidal saponins, flavonoids, flavanol glycosides, alkaloids, and tannins in varying quantities and proportions. These chemicals are thought to be physiologically active and are used in traditional communities for their medicinal properties. Mechanisms of action are not well understood, and may be mediated by changes in hormones, cytokines, and growth factors release, binding and action [61]. It may induce relaxation of the corpus cavernosum and therefore improve erectile function. It is proposed that saponins like dioscine, diosgenin, and protodioscin can have beneficial effects on libido [62].

Few studies have properly assessed the role of Tribulus terrestris in treating ED and HSDD in men, amid anecdotal claims of varying efficacy. A randomised double-blind, placebo-controlled trial was reported in 2016 across multiple sites in Bulgaria [63]. Patients were recruited from andrology, endocrinology and urology clinics and included males with ages >18 and <65 years, with mild to moderate ED, as defined by the IEFF score. Excluded patients were those with severe ED, spinal cord injury, primary HSDD, hyperprolactinaemia < two times upper limit, total testosterone < 8 mmol/l (230.7 ng/dl), uncontrolled major psychiatric disorders, chronic alcohol overuse, poorly controlled diabetes with HbA1c >7.0%, hypertension, unstable cardiovascular disease, stage 4 chronic kidney disease, elevated liver function tests > three times upper limit normal, prostate hypertrophy or cancer, or receiving androgen treatment. 180 patients were randomised to active group or a placebo-matched group. The active drug contained two tablets (500 mg) Tribestan administered orally three times daily after meals for 12 weeks. Tribestan (Sopharma AD) is a herbal medicinal product of Bulgaria origin, standardised with respect to furostanol saponins, calculated against protodioscin. Each tablet contains the active substance TT herba extractum siccum (35–45:1) 250 mg. The control group received identical tablet in colour and taste.

Patients were monitored monthly, with their sexual function assessed by the IIEF psychometric tool and the Global Efficacy Question (GEQ) log. Blood testing were performed at the start and end of the study and adverse events were carefully noted throughout and post study. The study showed that patients receiving Tribulus terrestris reported higher IIEF scores 2.70 OR (1.40–4.01) CI, and GEQ 4.55 OR (2.35–8.93) CI. These patients reported significantly improved erectile function, intercourse satisfaction, orgasmic function, sexual desire, and overall satisfaction. Over the course of treatment, patients receiving Tribulus terrestris did not exhibit differences in lipids, blood pressure, hormones such as total testosterone, free testosterone, SHBG, and dehydroepiandrosterone sulphate (DHEAS). Therefore, individuals with mild to moderate ED, may benefit from Tribulus terrestris without significant changes in lipids, and BP.

8.2 Selective androgen receptor modulators

As mentioned, testosterone exerts its main actions by binding to the AR, triggering important cellular signalling processes and gene transcriptions. It also has important secondary effects via aromatisation to estrogens, impacting on androgenic alopecia, bone re-modelling and by converting to DHT via 5α-reductase, exerting potent stimulatory effects on prostate growth. Since the 1990s, the concept of Selective Androgen Receptor Modulators (SARMs) as molecules that selectively activate ARs in targeted tissues without aromatisation to estrogens or undergoing 5α-reductase conversion to DHT is appealing [64]. SARMs can be engineered to specifically target AR in certain tissues while minimizing off-target effects. For example, SARMs would activate AR in muscle and bone, whilst sparing other tissues such as prostate, heart and liver. There is minimal variation in the AR structure, but the regulatory milieu of each tissue allows SARMs to possess relative tissue specificity. Upon entering the cell, SARMs bind to the AR in the cytosol, which dissociates from heat shock proteins and enters the nucleus, where the ligand-AR complex then binds with AR responsive peptides (co-activators or co-repressors) specific to certain tissues. This will influence how the SARM-AR complex may bind specific DNA sequences and lead to transcriptional regulation of androgen-responsive genes. Several experimental SARMs were available since 1998, with pre-clinical studies demonstrating positive effects on osteoporosis, cancer cachexia, and detrusor urinary incontinence. However, to date, they have not demonstrated enough efficacy or safety to pass the clinical trials [64]. Therefore at present, SARMs cannot be a substitute for managing androgen deficiency.

8.3 Estrogen antagonism

As mentioned afore, regulation of gonadotropin secretion occurs through stimulation by GnRH from the hypothalamus, and negative inhibition of the gonadotroph cells from testosterone and estrogens respectively. Selective Estrogen Receptor Modulators (SERM) work by selectively antagonising E2 receptors on the gonadotroph cells, abolishing the inhibition on gonadotropin release, and therefore elevate gonadotropins and testosterone levels. Likewise, by preventing the conversion of testosterone to oestradiol, aromatase inhibitors (AIs) block the inhibitory effect of oestradiol on hypothalamus and pituitary, thereby increasing LH-stimulated testosterone production. Estrogen antagonism is effective in normalising testosterone levels in men with functional hypogonadism [65–70], and both SERMs and AIs increase the testosterone/estrogen ratio with the latter, significantly more so.

The use of clomiphene citrate a SERM, was studied in obese males (<40 years) with total testosterone 10.4 nmol/l (<300 ng/dl) in a randomised double-blind placebo-controlled trial over 12 weeks. That showed positive findings with significantly improved erectile function, lean and muscle mass [71]. Use of SERMs may have beneficial effects on male fertility. Obese men aged 18–60 years with functional hypogonadism were randomised to receive enclomiphene, testosterone gel or placebo in a randomised double-blind double-dummy placebo-controlled trial over 16 weeks. Enclomiphene is a trans-isomer of clomiphene with consistent estrogen antagonism. As expected, there is a similar doubling of total testosterone levels in both treatment arms from a baseline of 7.0 nmol/l (203 ng/dl) but elevation of both FSH and LH levels in enclomiphene users and suppression in testosterone gel users. This was associated with a significant 80% increase in sperm concentration in men receiving enclomiphene, whilst the testosterone users showed 50% reduction [72]. An early study also suggested the possible benefit of addition of 400 mg daily vitamin E (an antioxidant) to clomiphene, in an RCT, which resulted in significant near-doubling of sperm counts and resulted in near tripling of pregnancies compared to placebo by 6 months [73].

The effect of anastrozole, a popular AI was compared with testosterone gel and placebo in older (>70 years) overweight men with functional hypogonadism using a 12-month RCT [68]. Both AI and T improved proximal muscle strength but not hand grip strength compared with placebo. Only the T group increased gait speed. There were increases in lean body mass and reduction in fat mass in the intervention groups (AI and T) but they were not statistically significant. An earlier 12-month RCT in 2009 comparing anastrozole and placebo did not observe significantly improved strength or muscle mass in older hypogonadal men receiving anastrozole. However, it may have resulted in improvement in quality of life as there was a documented reduction in ADAM scores, although the statistical significance was not reported [74]. There are variable effects and conflicting reports on sperm count and motility. It is possible that some level of estrogenic activity may be necessary for FSH stimulation and therefore sperm production [75]. Unfortunately, an RCT comparing clomiphene and anastrozole in obese younger males (mean age 32–33 years) failed to find any significance in improved quality of life outcomes using ADAM or IIEF scores, or improved sperm characteristics [70].

Risk of venous thromboembolism (VTE) taking SERMs is 0.12% per year in the normal population but likely at least three times elevated in patients with cancer. The risks of VTE in AIs are considerably less than SERMs and may be similar to that of the general population [70]. However, the overall risk may be increased in the elderly and those with cardiovascular risk factors [76]. Use of anastrozole in older men has been associated with statistically reduced lumbar spine bone density of >80% after 12 months, whilst those on testosterone gel have preserved bone density [68]. SERMs are known to increase bone mineral density [67]. An advantage of estrogen antagonists such as SERMs and AIs is that they tend to be safer in estrogen-sensitive cancers such as hepatocellular, and prostate cancers, and are often used for male breast cancer treatment. Burnett-Bowie et al. found that the PSA levels in older men receiving anastrozole were not different to placebo, despite the substantial increase in testosterone levels. It is possible the reduction of intra-prostate estrogen levels offer protection [74].

9. Conclusion

Testosterone substitution or replacement therapy is effective for managing testosterone deficiency. Popular routes of administration include oral, transdermal, and intramuscular. Scrotal application of testosterone cream is recently made available. Physician's choice of one preparation over another is based on testosterone bioavailability, side effect profile and ability to achieve therapeutic levels. Patient's choice is influenced by comfort, ease of use and product acceptability. This is important for compliance and achievement of good outcomes. Testosterone replacement can be overused and associated with adverse effects. Individuals at risk are older, obese with chronic cardiorespiratory disorders, and lower urinary tract symptoms. Therapeutic monitoring is vital and is achieved through measuring serum testosterone levels and clinical follow-up. Decision on therapy outcomes should be individualised, based on symptom control and testosterone effects on organ function. Supra-therapeutic testosterone levels should be avoided as adverse outcomes such as worsening obstructive sleep apnoea, polycythaemia, and prostatic growth stimulation are more likely. Assessment of symptomatic improvement is important to justify the risks versus benefits of ongoing testosterone therapy. Dose adjustment should be individualised, accounting for the patients' co-morbidity profile, testosterone levels, haematocrit, and PSA levels. Assessment of osteoporosis with baseline bone mineral density is important, and a progress bone mineral density assessment in 12–24 months may be useful to document benefit or lack thereof. Above all, patients must always be counselled on holistic and self-care management, and include healthy lifestyle measures, such as smoking cessation, and weight management. Non-testosterone substitution options offer alternatives to testosterone therapy, and may have some positive benefit, but are not generally considered as mainstream therapy at the moment.

Author details

Kenneth W.K. Ho
Faculty of Medicine and Health Sciences, Macquarie University, Sydney, Australia

*Address all correspondence to: kenneth.ho@mq.edu.au

References

[1] Hayes FJ, DeCruz S, Seminara SB, Boepple PA, Crowley WF Jr. Differential regulation of gonadotropin secretion by testosterone in the human male: Absence of a negative feedback effect of testosterone on follicle-stimulating hormone secretion. The Journal of Clinical Endocrinology and Metabolism. 2001;**86**(1):53-58

[2] Negro-Vilar A. Selective androgen receptor modulators (SARMs): A novel approach to androgen therapy for the new millennium. The Journal of Clinical Endocrinology and Metabolism. 1999;**84**(10):3459-3462

[3] Pirog EC, Collins DC. Metabolism of dihydrotestosterone in human liver: Importance of 3alpha- and 3beta-hydroxysteroid dehydrogenase. The Journal of Clinical Endocrinology and Metabolism. 1999;**84**(9):3217-3221

[4] Naamneh Elzenaty R, du Toit T, Fluck CE. Basics of androgen synthesis and action. Best Practice & Research. Clinical Endocrinology & Metabolism. 2022;**101665**

[5] Yeap BB, Alfonso H, Chubb SA, Handelsman DJ, Hankey GJ, Norman PE, et al. Reference ranges and determinants of testosterone, dihydrotestosterone, and estradiol levels measured using liquid chromatography-tandem mass spectrometry in a population-based cohort of older men. Journal of Clinical Endocrinology and Metabolism. 2012;**97**(11):4030-4039

[6] Grossmann M, Anawalt BD, Wu FC. Clinical practice patterns in the assessment and management of low testosterone in men: An international survey of endocrinologists. Clinical Endocrinology. 2015;**82**(2):234-241

[7] Snyder PJ, Bhasin S, Cunningham GR, Matsumoto AM, Stephens-Shields AJ, Cauley JA, et al. Effects of testosterone treatment in older men. The New England Journal of Medicine. 2016;**374**(7):611-624

[8] Haider KS, Haider A, Saad F, Doros G, Hanefeld M, Dhindsa S, et al. Remission of type 2 diabetes following long-term treatment with injectable testosterone undecanoate in patients with hypogonadism and type 2 diabetes: 11-year data from a real-world registry study. Diabetes, Obesity & Metabolism. 2020;**22**(11):2055-2068

[9] Wittert G, Bracken K, Robledo KP, Grossmann M, Yeap BB, Handelsman DJ, et al. Testosterone treatment to prevent or revert type 2 diabetes in men enrolled in a lifestyle programme (T4DM): A randomised, double-blind, placebo-controlled, 2-year, phase 3b trial. Lancet Diabetes and Endocrinology. 2021;**9**(1):32-45

[10] Mohamed O, Freundlich RE, Dakik HK, Grober ED, Najari B, Lipshultz LI, et al. The quantitative ADAM questionnaire: A new tool in quantifying the severity of hypogonadism. International Journal of Impotence Research. 2010;**22**(1):20-24

[11] Rosen RC, Cappelleri JC, Smith MD, Lipsky J, Pena BM. Development and evaluation of an abridged, 5-item version of the International Index of Erectile Function (IIEF-5) as a diagnostic tool for erectile dysfunction. International Journal of Impotence Research. 1999;**11**(6):319-326

[12] van Londen GJ, Levy ME, Perera S, Nelson JB, Greenspan SL. Body composition changes during androgen deprivation therapy for prostate cancer:

A 2-year prospective study. Critical Reviews in Oncology/Hematology. 2008;**68**(2):172-177

[13] Katznelson L, Finkelstein JS, Schoenfeld DA, Rosenthal DI, Anderson EJ, Klibanski A. Increase in bone density and lean body mass during testosterone administration in men with acquired hypogonadism. Journal of Clinical Endocrinology and Metabolism. 1996;**81**(12):4358-4365

[14] Huang LT, Wang JH. The therapeutic intervention of sex steroid hormones for sarcopenia. Frontiers in Medicine. 2021;**8**:739251

[15] Ebeling PR. Clinical practice. Osteoporosis in men. The New England Journal of Medicine. 2008;**358**(14):1474-1482

[16] Greenspan SL, Coates P, Sereika SM, Nelson JB, Trump DL, Resnick NM. Bone loss after initiation of androgen deprivation therapy in patients with prostate cancer. Journal of Clinical Endocrinology and Metabolism. 2005;**90**(12):6410-6417

[17] Batrinos ML. Testosterone and aggressive behavior in man. International Journal of Endocrinology and Metabolism. 2012;**10**(3):563-568

[18] Wang C, Alexander G, Berman N, Salehian B, Davidson T, McDonald V, et al. Testosterone replacement therapy improves mood in hypogonadal men – a clinical research center study. Journal of Clinical Endocrinology and Metabolism. 1996;**81**(10):3578-3583

[19] Hoberman JM, Yesalis CE. The history of synthetic testosterone. Scientific American. 1995;**272**(2):76-81

[20] Foss GL. A comparison of the relative efficacy of methyltestosterone by the gastric and oral transmucosal routes. Journal of Endocrinology. 1956;**13**(3):269-273

[21] Foss GL, Simpson SL. Oral methyltestosterone and jaundice. British Medical Journal. 1959;**1**(5117):259-263

[22] Bagatell CJ, Bremner WJ. Androgens in men – uses and abuses. The New England Journal of Medicine. 1996;**334**(11):707-714

[23] Behre HM, Nieschlag E. Testosterone preparations for clinical use in males. In: Nieschlag E, Behre HM, Nieschlag S, editors. Testosterone: Action, Deficiency, Substitution. 4th ed. United Kingdom: Cambridge University Press; 2012. pp. 309-335

[24] Nieschlag E, Cuppers HJ, Wiegelmann W, Wickings EJ. Bioavailability and LH-suppressing effect of different testosterone preparations in normal and hypogonadal men. Hormone Research. 1976;**7**(3):138-145

[25] Nieschlag E, Nieschlag S. Testosterone deficiency: a historical perspective. Asian Journal of Andrology. 2014;**16**(2):161-168

[26] Snyder PJ, Lawrence DA. Treatment of male hypogonadism with testosterone enanthate. Journal of Clinical Endocrinology and Metabolism. 1980;**51**(6):1335-1339

[27] Salmimies P, Kockott G, Pirke KM, Vogt HJ, Schill WB. Effects of testosterone replacement on sexual behavior in hypogonadal men. Archives of Sexual Behavior. 1982;**11**(4):345-353

[28] Nankin HR. Hormone kinetics after intramuscular testosterone cypionate. Fertility and Sterility. 1987;**47**(6):1004-1009

[29] Skakkebaek NE, Bancroft J, Davidson DW, Warner P. Androgen replacement with oral testosterone undecanoate in hypogonadal men: A double blind controlled study. Clinical Endocrinology. 1981;**14**(1):49-61

[30] Horst HJ, Holtje WJ, Dennis M, Coert A, Geelen J, Voigt KD. Lymphatic absorption and metabolism of orally administered testosterone undecanoate in man. Klinische Wochenschrift. 1976;**54**(18):875-879

[31] Zhang GY, Gu YQ, Wang XH, Cui YG, Bremner WJ. A pharmacokinetic study of injectable testosterone undecanoate in hypogonadal men. Journal of Andrology. 1998;**19**(6):761-768

[32] Corona G, Maseroli E, Maggi M. Injectable testosterone undecanoate for the treatment of hypogonadism. Expert Opinion on Pharmacotherapy. 2014;**15**(13):1903-1926

[33] Nieschlag E, Buchter D, Von Eckardstein S, Abshagen K, Simoni M, Behre HM. Repeated intramuscular injections of testosterone undecanoate for substitution therapy in hypogonadal men. Clinical Endocrinology. 1999;**51**(6):757-763

[34] Wang C, Harnett M, Dobs AS, Swerdloff RS. Pharmacokinetics and safety of long-acting testosterone undecanoate injections in hypogonadal men: an 84-week phase III clinical trial. Journal of Andrology. 2010;**31**(5):457-465

[35] Handelsman DJ, Mackey MA, Howe C, Turner L, Conway AJ. An analysis of testosterone implants for androgen replacement therapy. Clinical Endocrinology. 1997;**47**(3):311-316

[36] Jockenhovel F, Vogel E, Kreutzer M, Reinhardt W, Lederbogen S, Reinwein D. Pharmacokinetics and pharmacodynamics of subcutaneous testosterone implants in hypogonadal men. Clinical Endocrinology. 1996;**45**(1):61-71

[37] Jungwirth A, Plas E, Geurts P. Clinical experience with Andriol Testocaps – the first Austrian surveillance study on the treatment of late-onset hypogonadism. The Aging Male. 2007;**10**(4):183-187

[38] Wang C, Swerdloff R, Kipnes M, Matsumoto AM, Dobs AS, Cunningham G, et al. New testosterone buccal system (Striant) delivers physiological testosterone levels: Pharmacokinetics study in hypogonadal men. Journal of Clinical Endocrinology and Metabolism. 2004;**89**(8):3821-3829

[39] Findlay JC, Place VA, Snyder PJ. Transdermal delivery of testosterone. Journal of Clinical Endocrinology and Metabolism. 1987;**64**(2):266-268

[40] Meikle AW, Mazer NA, Moellmer JF, Stringham JD, Tolman KG, Sanders SW, et al. Enhanced transdermal delivery of testosterone across nonscrotal skin produces physiological concentrations of testosterone and its metabolites in hypogonadal men. Journal of Clinical Endocrinology and Metabolism. 1992;**74**(3):623-628

[41] Yu Z, Gupta SK, Hwang SS, Cook DM, Duckett MJ, Atkinson LE. Transdermal testosterone administration in hypogonadal men: Comparison of pharmacokinetics at different sites of application and at the first and fifth days of application. Journal of Clinical Pharmacology. 1997;**37**(12):1129-1138

[42] Yu Z, Gupta SK, Hwang SS, Kipnes MS, Mooradian AD, Snyder PJ, et al. Testosterone pharmacokinetics after application of an investigational transdermal system in hypogonadal

men. Journal of Clinical Pharmacology. 1997;**37**(12):1139-1145

[43] Wang C, Swerdloff RS, Iranmanesh A, Dobs A, Snyder PJ, Cunningham G, et al. Transdermal testosterone gel improves sexual function, mood, muscle strength, and body composition parameters in hypogonadal men. Journal of Clinical Endocrinology and Metabolism. 2000;**85**(8):2839-2853

[44] Wang C, Ilani N, Arver S, McLachlan RI, Soulis T, Watkinson A. Efficacy and safety of the 2% formulation of testosterone topical solution applied to the axillae in androgen-deficient men. Clinical Endocrinology. 2011;**75**(6):836-843

[45] Wittert GA, Harrison RW, Buckley MJ, Wlodarczyk J. An open-label, phase 2, single centre, randomized, crossover design bioequivalence study of AndroForte 5 testosterone cream and Testogel 1% testosterone gel in hypogonadal men: study LP101. Andrology. 2016;**4**(1):41-45

[46] Iyer R, Mok SF, Savkovic S, Turner L, Fraser G, Desai R, et al. Pharmacokinetics of testosterone cream applied to scrotal skin. Andrology. 2017;**5**(4):725-731

[47] Gronski MA, Grober ED, Gottesman IS, Ormsby RW, Bryson N. Efficacy of nasal testosterone gel (Natesto®) stratified by baseline endogenous testosterone levels. Journal of the Endocrine Society. 2019;**3**(9):1652-1662

[48] Lee J, Brock G, Barkin J, Bryson N, Gronski MA, Ormsby R. The My-T study: patient satisfaction and preference comparing topical and nasal testosterone therapies. Canadian Urological Association Journal. 2019:384-389

[49] Wilson JD, Griffin JE. The use and misuse of androgens. Metabolism. 1980;**29**(12):1278-1295

[50] Conway AJ, Boylan LM, Howe C, Ross G, Handelsman DJ. Randomized clinical trial of testosterone replacement therapy in hypogonadal men. International Journal of Andrology. 1988;**11**(4):247-264

[51] Yesalis CE, Anderson WA, Buckley WE, Wright JE. Incidence of the nonmedical use of anabolic-androgenic steroids. NIDA Research Monograph. 1990;**102**:97-112

[52] Wood RI, Stanton SJ. Testosterone and sport: Current perspectives. Hormones and Behavior. 2012;**61**(1):147-155

[53] Giorgi A, Weatherby RP, Murphy PW. Muscular strength, body composition and health responses to the use of testosterone enanthate: A double blind study. Journal of Science and Medicine in Sport. 1999;**2**(4):341-355

[54] Buckley WE, Yesalis CE 3rd, Friedl KE, Anderson WA, Streit AL, Wright JE. Estimated prevalence of anabolic steroid use among male high school seniors. Journal of the American Medical Association. 1988;**260**(23):3441-3445

[55] Ho KWK. Opioid-induced androgen deficiency (OPIAD): Prevalence, consequence, and efficacy of testosterone replacement. Current Opin in Endo and Metab Res. 2019;**6**:54-59

[56] Hembree WC, Cohen-Kettenis PT, Gooren L, Hannema SE, Meyer WJ, Murad MH, et al. Endocrine treatment of gender-dysphoric/gender-incongruent persons: An endocrine society clinical practice guideline. Journal of Clinical

Endocrinology and Metabolism. 2017;**102**(11):3869-3903

[57] Pelusi C, Costantino A, Martelli V, Lambertini M, Bazzocchi A, Ponti F, et al. Effects of three different testosterone formulations in female-to-male transsexual persons. Journal of Sexual Medicine. 2014;**11**(12):3002-3011

[58] Asscheman H, Giltay EJ, Megens JA, de Ronde WP, van Trotsenburg MA, Gooren LJ. A long-term follow-up study of mortality in transsexuals receiving treatment with cross-sex hormones. European Journal of Endocrinology. 2011;**164**(4):635-642

[59] Stancampiano MR, Lucas-Herald AK, Russo G, Rogol AD, Ahmed SF. Testosterone therapy in adolescent boys: The need for a structured approach. Hormone Research in Pædiatrics. 2019;**92**(4):215-228

[60] Pok S, Barn VA, Wong HJ, Blackburn AC, Board P, Farrell GC, et al. Testosterone regulation of cyclin E kinase: A key factor in determining gender differences in hepatocarcinogenesis. Journal of Gastroenterology and Hepatology. 2016;**31**(6):1210-1219

[61] Sirotkin AV, Kolesarova A. Puncture vine (*Tribulus terrestris* L.) in control of health and reproduction. Physiological Research. 2021;**70**(Suppl4):S657-SS67

[62] Sellami M, Slimeni O, Pokrywka A, Kuvacic G, Hayes LD, Milic M, et al. Herbal medicine for sports: A review. Journal of the International Society of Sports Nutrition. 2018;**15**:14

[63] Kamenov Z, Fileva S, Kalinov K, Jannini EA. Evaluation of the efficacy and safety of *Tribulus terrestris* in male sexual dysfunction - a prospective, randomized, double-blind, placebo-controlled clinical trial. Maturitas. 2017;**99**:20-26

[64] Narayanan R, Coss CC, Dalton JT. Development of selective androgen receptor modulators (SARMs). Molecular and Cellular Endocrinology. 2018;**465**:134-142

[65] Patel DP, Brant WO, Myers JB, Presson AP, Johnstone EB, Dorais JA, et al. The safety and efficacy of clomiphene citrate in hypoandrogenic and subfertile men. International Journal of Impotence Research. 2015;**27**(6):221-224

[66] Pelusi C, Giagulli VA, Baccini M, Fanelli F, Mezzullo M, Fazzini A, et al. Clomiphene citrate effect in obese men with low serum testosterone treated with metformin due to dysmetabolic disorders: A randomized, double-blind, placebo-controlled study. PLoS One. 2017;**12**(9):e0183369

[67] Wong SK, Mohamad NV, Jayusman PA, Shuid AN, Ima-Nirwana S, Chin KY. The use of selective estrogen receptor modulators on bone health in men. The Aging Male. 2019;**22**(2):89-101

[68] Awouters M, Vanderschueren D, Antonio L. Aromatase inhibitors and selective estrogen receptor modulators: Unconventional therapies for functional hypogonadism? Andrology. 2020;**8**(6):1590-1597

[69] Dias JP, Melvin D, Simonsick EM, Carlson O, Shardell MD, Ferrucci L, et al. Effects of aromatase inhibition vs. testosterone in older men with low testosterone: randomized-controlled trial. Andrology. 2016;**4**(1):33-40

[70] Helo S, Ellen J, Mechlin C, Feustel P, Grossman M, Ditkoff E, et al. A randomized prospective double-blind comparison trial of clomiphene citrate

and anastrozole in raising testosterone in hypogonadal infertile men. Journal of Sexual Medicine. 2015;**12**(8):1761-1769

[71] Soares AH, Horie NC, Chiang LAP, Caramelli B, Matheus MG, Campos AH, et al. Effects of clomiphene citrate on male obesity-associated hypogonadism: A randomized, double-blind, placebo-controlled study. International Journal of Obesity. 2018;**42**(5):953-963

[72] Kim ED, McCullough A, Kaminetsky J. Oral enclomiphene citrate raises testosterone and preserves sperm counts in obese hypogonadal men, unlike topical testosterone: restoration instead of replacement. BJU International. 2016;**117**(4):677-685

[73] Ghanem H, Shaeer O, El-Segini A. Combination clomiphene citrate and antioxidant therapy for idiopathic male infertility: A randomized controlled trial. Fertility and Sterility. 2010;**93**(7):2232-2235

[74] Burnett-Bowie SA, Roupenian KC, Dere ME, Lee H, Leder BZ. Effects of aromatase inhibition in hypogonadal older men: A randomized, double-blind, placebo-controlled trial. Clinical Endocrinology. 2009;**70**(1):116-123

[75] O'Donnell L, Robertson KM, Jones ME, Simpson ER. Estrogen and spermatogenesis. Endocrine Reviews. 2001;**22**(3):289-318

[76] Lycette JL, Luoh SW, Beer TM, Deloughery TG. Acute bilateral pulmonary emboli occurring while on adjuvant aromatase inhibitor therapy with anastrozole: Case report and review of the literature. Breast Cancer Research and Treatment. 2006;**99**(3):249-255